ELEVATE YOUR ENERGY

ELEVATE YOUR ENERGY

THE MOST INSPIRING WAY TO TAKE YOUR ENERGY TO THE NEXT LEVEL

Foreword by Dr John Demartini
Human Behaviour Specialist, Educator & Teacher From 'The Secret'

Disclaimer

All the information, techniques, skills and concepts contained within this publication are of the nature of general comment only and are not in any way recommended as individual advice. The intent is to offer a variety of information to provide a wider range of choices now and in the future, recognising that we all have widely diverse circumstances and viewpoints.

Should any reader choose to make use of the information contained herein, this is their decision, and the contributors (and their companies), authors and publishers do not assume any responsibilities whatsoever under any condition or circumstances. It is recommended that the reader obtain their own independent advice.

First Edition 2021

NATIONAL LIBRARY OF AUSTRALIA

A catalogue record for this book is available from the National Library of Australia

Creator: Harvey, Benjamin J., author.
Other Authors:
Austen, Karen | Galipo, Veronica | Morley, Karen | Peck, Elise | Peebles, Andrea| Rei, Marina |Reynolds, Robyn | Shanahan, Leonie

Title: Elevate your Energy / Benjamin J Harvey.

ISBN: 9781925471526 (paperback)

Published by Author Express
www.AuthorExpress.com
publish@authorexpress.com

Dedication

To fellow learners wanting to take their energy to the next level. This book is dedicated to you.

Benjamin J Harvey and co-authors

Foreword by Dr John Demartini

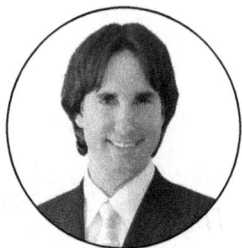

For over forty eight years I have studied the art, science and philosophy of wellness and numerous natural healing arts, particularly in relation to the mind-body connection. I have my doctorate in chiropractic, and I have specialized studies in the integrated fields of physiology, psychology and philosophy.

One subfield that I was blessed to do more extensive research in, was axiology, which is the study of value and worth. Every human being lives by a set of priorities or hierarchy of values, and no two people have the same set or series. For each individual their set of values is truly unique as are their fingerprints and retinal patterns. Their individual world is filtered through their unique hierarchy of values, which determines how they perceive, what they decide and how they act.

Whatever is highest on your set of values is what you're most eager to learn and most spontaneously inspired to act upon from within. No one needs to remind you to get up in the morning and do what you love most. You just love doing it. On the other hand, you procrastinate and hesitate on your lowest values and require outside motivation.

The hierarchy of your values and the impact they have on your perceptions also affects your physiology. In other words, how your body functions. The way you perceive your world affects your energy levels, your cell functions, your genetic expressions and your overall physical condition.

Your psychology underlies your physiology and therefore plays a vital role in your various health conditions. Your body provides feedback, in the form of symptoms, that guide you to be your most congruent, authentic and inspired self, and helps you live a more fulfilling highest value based life.

Basically, if you're not living congruently or in accordance with your true highest values, you're going to experience a lower energy level and manifest illness within the body. It's well-known that your imbalanced perceptions and their resultant emotions - anger, feelings of loss or grief and other states of distress, can run down your immune system and lead to various illnesses, including cancer, while higher priority based love and appreciation can lead you back to wellness.

Your overall vitality is proportionate to the clarity of your highest value based mission and vision. You will experience the most vibrant life when you are living according to your highest values congruently and authentically. When you live according to your highest values, you're rewarded physiologically with increased energy and psychologically with poise, presence and meaningful and purposeful action.

Throughout this book, you will find healers and coaches with various methodologies, all ultimately working to bring your body back to psychological and physiological homeostasis. A therapist, facilitator or healer who works from an authentic and congruent space of love and gratitude of the heart, and certainty and presence of the mind, will affect some form of healing in almost anyone with whom they come in contact. Every healing art has a place in the great field of wellness and every healing modality and treatment can be of service - though it's important to realise that all true wellness starts in the mind and works through the heart in both the healer and the healed.

You can be a master of your destiny or a victim of your history by living according to your highest or lower values. When you go to bed thankful, you wake up with more inspiration and are more likely to take command of your destiny and bring about healing from within and about.

Being grateful, which spontaneously occurs more frequently when you are living congruently, will Elevate Your Energy and transform your mind and body. It causes your heart to open and allows your feelings of love to flow, and love and gratitude are the two greatest healers in life.

Dr John F. Demartini
Human Behaviour Specialist
www.DrDemartini.com

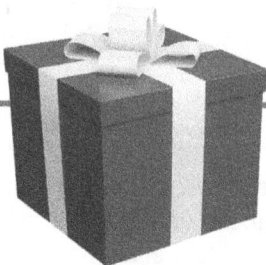

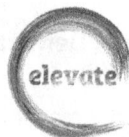

Contents

"Giving yourself permission
to do what you love is the key to
elevating all areas of your life."

~ Benjamin J Harvey

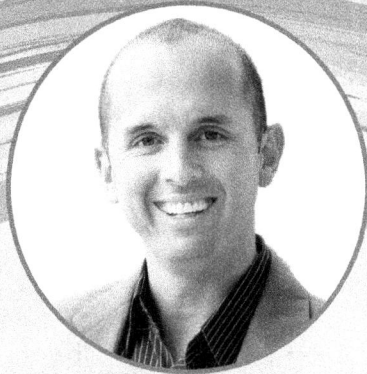

Benjamin J Harvey

Live Your Love

For over a decade, Benjamin J Harvey has studied the psychology of empowerment to help people find the answer to life's most intriguing questions.

Knowing that books like the Elevate series empowers individuals to bring their dreams into reality, Benjamin has assisted thousands of people across the globe to invest in themselves by showing how they can live their dream.

In 2009, he founded Authentic Education with business partner Cham Tang, to help empower people to live abundantly on purpose. As a result, Authentic Education went on to achieve something that has never been done before in the history of personal development. They received the BRW Fast Starters Award in 2013 and then backed it up in 2015 by being named in the BRW Fast 100 as the thirty-eighth fastest-growing company in Australia.

Having delivered well over 10,000 one-on-one coaching sessions, and training thousands of people across the globe, Ben now specializes in guiding people in how they can make a difference by achieving success doing what they love.

Ben has been featured on The Today Show in the Sydney Morning Herald and on ABC Radio.

Benjamin J Harvey

Live Your Love

What's your top tip for someone to elevate their energy?

It's simple! Do what you love. First and foremost, people need to listen to their heart and have the courage to follow their inner voice that already knows what they're here to do.

People who do what they love can't wait to get up in the morning and have all the energy in the world to work on things that are valuable to them.

Every day, I hear about people going to jobs they hate. They're suffering from *Mondayitis* and live for getting through hump day. Often, it's because they don't know there's another way to live. Or maybe they've spent so much time and money obtaining a degree at university, they feel they need to continue in that role for the rest of their life. Other times there's pressure to follow in the tracks of their parents and be a doctor or lawyer, and along the way they forgot to follow their own authentic dreams.

I would choose doing what you love any day of the week over how much money you earn. There are many types of currency in life, and money is only one of them. I've had so many professionals coming through my academy who've had a successful career and now want to explore what they really, truly want to do, rather than what their goals were when they started their career twenty years ago or more.

Most people spend a third of their time at work, so therefore one of your highest priorities in life should be finding happiness and fulfilment in your career. The other two thirds are occupied with sleeping and recreation time.

How can someone find their purpose in life?

There's so much pressure on people these days to find their passion and purpose. They're waiting for that *aha* moment or light bulb to go off to know for certain they're on their path.

I'd like to take the pressure off by saying your purpose can change at different times in your life, so just knowing you can have more than one is often a relief. The next is that you need to actually go out and try new things.

One of the most common questions I'm asked is, "Do I really need absolute certainty about what my purpose is before taking the necessary actions to live the most fulfilling life possible?"

My answer is always, "You don't have to be certain about what you're going to do in life!"

In fact, you can be as unclear as humanly possible, yet still take the necessary actions that will allow you to be fulfilled.

Sitting at home wanting to be crystal clear as to your purpose in life is as insane as refusing to date anybody until you're certain you're in love, fully committed to spending the rest of your life with them.

Guess what? We've all been there before. Millions of people around the world are going through this process right now:

- They're sitting at a job they don't like.
- They're doing activities that aren't fulfilling.
- They're making just enough money to barely pay the bills, so they can go back to something they don't enjoy.

The reason they're doing this is because they've been sold a lie that until you have total conviction about what your next step should be, you can't take it.

People always say to me, "Ben, what's it like knowing with absolute certainty what you're going to dedicate your life to?"

I have to tell them I don't even know what that means. I have no idea.

All I know is that right now, talking to you is inspiring to me. Sharing this information with you to help you feel liberated and experience freedom in your life, inspires me. I will tell you that if I wake up tomorrow, and this doesn't inspire me anymore, I'm not going to do it anymore.

One of the greatest lessons I ever got from one of my spiritual teachers was this:

"Just because you manifest something, doesn't mean you have to use it."

So even if you've created the most successful coaching practice you could, it doesn't mean that if you started loving property management, you'd have to keep doing coaching.

How do you start your day?

I'm a big fan of meditation, and I believe that five to twenty minutes of good meditation in the morning is always going to put you in a great position to have more emotional control.

So in the morning, when I first wake up, I lie in bed with my eyes closed and imagine my events full of people, my daughter's good health, my wife's good health, my family having a great life, my business growing and all of us travelling together. I imagine everything I love in my life exactly the way I want it. Then I do some basic gentle awareness of my breath from five to twenty minutes. It's a simple and easy way to start my day.

What is The Gap?

Voluntary choice has a huge impact on your happiness. The problem is, you don't typically have a lot of time between what life throws at you and how you respond to it.

But there's a way you can have a voluntary choice. Please refer to the simple diagram below.

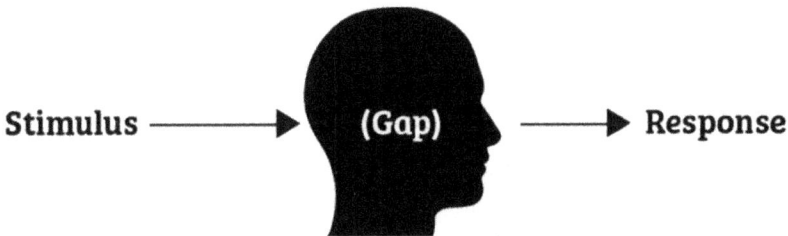

Stimulus ⟶ (Gap) ⟶ Response

As you can see, there's point one, which is the stimulus, and point two is the response. So in point one, you yell at someone, and in point two they yell back. The gap between you yelling at someone and them getting angry and yelling back, equals how much voluntary choice you have.

Now in life, it's nanoseconds. For instance, you get cut off, and you honk your horn. You didn't choose this response. There was no volunteering. It was a nanosecond. The reason is because fifty percent of your programming said, "That person was rude. Honk your horn."

When you speak to yogis, they will talk about this thing called the gap. You want to meditate? Enter the gap. You want to be spiritual? Enter the gap. You want to have a better life? Enter the gap.

The gap is the distance between stimulus and response. The bigger the gap, the greater your voluntary choice. The smaller the gap, the less your voluntary choice. That's it. If you want to have a happier life, all you have to do is extend the gap between these two points.

How can someone extend The Gap?

Extending the gap requires practice that comes in the form of meditation. There are many different meditating techniques, and none are better or worse than the others. All I'm interested in is if the meditation works.

I meet a lot of people who've been meditating for years, and there's still no gap between stimulus and response. None. They'll say, "Well, I've been meditating for forty years, and I had this incredible ... Shut up! I'm freaking talking! Anyway, I'm so Zen. I'm just totally into peace". It's like, why do they bother meditating? It's obviously not working. Stop it.

Remember, it's not that you know so much, it's that you know so much that isn't so. Most people who think they're meditating are not. They're doing guided imagery healing (GIH), which doesn't assist you in having a gap between stimulus and response. It helps you become relaxed, yes, but not in creating the gap.

A lot of people listen to these CDs of a river running down pebbles as they're told they're sitting in a forest where hooded wise people come around and shine their light on them, and then they float up and fly around. I love those. I do them all the time, but I'm not ignorant enough to believe that's meditation, because if this is all you do, I hate to tell you, but your gap is only getting smaller.

This is because guided imagery healing makes you super aware of everything. Now, if you're way more in tune with your environment, you're getting triggered way more than everybody else. This means if you don't match awareness with balance, you're in all sorts of trouble.

Twenty years later, after all of this supposed meditation, these people aren't any more emotionally in control than they were before. That's because to make it more marketable, they called it guided meditation, when it was really guided imagery healing.

If all you do is awareness-based activities, you'll be more agitated than ever before and make connections that don't exist, while not understanding why the other person isn't making them as well.

Or maybe you study a different type of meditation, where it's all about balance. You stare at a candle and don't move for hours. This method will make you fully balanced, but you'll have no awareness.

I've had many different meditation teachers. One of them is a gentleman by the name of S.N. Goenkam. He does *Vipassana* meditation and described it as being like the wings of a butterfly, with one being balance and the other awareness. He says they have to be equal in strength and size, or they can't fly. So if you only work on your balance, your gap is too big to be aware of anything, and if all you concentrate on is awareness, your gap is too small to be attuned to anything.

The perfect balance of these two is meditation. A lot of people use guided imagery for escapism, because for that one hour while they're down at their running nook, they're escaping life, and they feel better. But that doesn't transform any of the neurological pathways in the mind to help deal with that crappy stuff when the guided imagination process is over, because they're not building and expanding their gap.

There's a saying that a mind once stretched, can never go back to its original dimensions. Or, as Wayne Dyer used to say, "A set of Speedos once stretched, will never go back to their original dimensions".

So you learn a little bit of information and expand your mind, and then maybe you pick up a book, apply a little bit and expand your mind. Then you attend a seminar and expand it even more. When you start off with a small consciousness and keep stretching it until your world gets bigger, you'll start to believe you have a pretty expansive consciousness.

Meditation puts a massive gap between the stimulus and how you choose to respond. The bigger the gap, the more you get to voluntarily choose how you feel, which probably wouldn't include resentment, disgust, furiousness or complete body-numbing anger.

But if you don't have a gap, you can't make the choice.

How does meditation work?

I want to explain meditation to you in a way you'll get it, because a lot of people meditate but don't know what they're doing, which means they aren't really meditating.

The beautiful thing about meditation is that there's no delay. It's the most instantly gratifying technique you can do on planet Earth, and the benefits last, on average, about twenty-four hours.

Meditators activate the executive function, which is when eight specific functions in the brain all switch on at once to help you manifest what you want as if out of thin air. They are:

- impulse control
- organisation
- self-monitoring
- emotional control
- flexibility
- working memory
- task initiation
- planning and prioritisation.

The reason meditators seem to have the ability to synchronistically put things together and perceive events before they happen, is due to a heightened executive function. It looks magical, but it's only the brain doing what it's meant to be doing.

How can meditation be used to slow the aging process?

Mystical events do occur when you meditate, but if you forget about this for a second and just look at meditation in a scientific light, you'll see something miraculous.

I've sought answers at the anti-aging clinic, where they do extensive research on what stops people from aging. Basically, there are three chemicals in the body that if you know how to regulate, increase or reduce them, you can age way more slowly than everybody else.

1. DHEA

DHEA is a steroid hormone that your body naturally produces. It is a precursor to other hormones including testosterone and estrogen. It is also important in other bodily functions associated with mood, energy levels, executive function and memory. DHEA levels naturally lower as you age and people with medical conditions such as chronic fatigue syndrome seem to have a reduction in DHEA inside their system.

It has been discovered that when someone meditates, they can increase DHEA anywhere from 44 to 90 percent. That's pretty amazing. Having an adequate production of DHEA may assist a variety of bodily functions in slowing down the aging process.

2. Melatonin

What also happens when you meditate is that you produce a substance called melatonin. Production may increase anywhere from 100 to 300 percent, which means you feel more rested, and don't have to sleep as much, because you're not as lethargic.

Now, if you produce melatonin while you're meditating, it means the body perceives it's resting more than it is, and if that's the case, you don't age as much. Because if you want to quicken the aging process, try sleeping less. Reduce your sleep to two hours a night, and watch how fast you age. You can look in the mirror and see it happen. If you meditate to increase that melatonin, and trick the system into believing it's sleeping more than it is, then it may have an impact on aging.

3. Cortisol

Cortisol is great to have in your system. A lot of people say you need to get rid of it, but you don't. You need cortisol. You just don't require a lot of it, and most people have more than is necessary. Cortisol does affect blood pressure and a whole range of activities, but generally when you get stressed out, your cortisol levels increase.

A twenty-minute meditation in the morning may reduce cortisol production by 50 percent. That is, you can potentially halve your cortisol by meditating.

Here's another interesting fact. Researchers biologically tested meditators and non-meditators, and found that a non-meditator, on average, is about two to three years older than their biological age, while a meditator is twelve years *younger* than their biological age.

There's no reason not to meditate. It doesn't even have to be a spiritual practice if you don't want it to be. It's just a way of getting more out of your brain and your body.

How does meditation affect the brain cycle?

If while hooked up to an EEG machine, you were observed as you demonstrated certain behaviours, you would discover that your brain has different cycles.

When a song gets stuck in your head, you must have realised that the only way to get it out is to go to sleep. This is because as you awaken, your mind changes the cycles per second at which it's spinning.

As you slowly wake up, your brain gets faster and faster. This is when you're in beta, which consists of high frequency, low amplitude brainwaves that are involved in conscious thought and logical thinking, and tend to have a stimulating effect. Having the right amount allows you to focus and complete tasks easily. Alpha waves bridge the gap between your conscious thinking and subconscious mind, or the beta and theta. They help calm you down when necessary and promote feelings of deep relaxation.

So when you first wake up in the morning, instead of getting out of bed, hold your posture and meditate for five minutes. Don't move a muscle, even when your nose starts itching or your knee feels like it's going to explode and smash into a billion pieces. No matter what stimulus gets thrown at you, don't respond. This is how your body will understand you're in control of it.

After a couple of days of doing this, the body will work out that unless the mind says you can do it, you can't. If you're able to sit there without moving and avoid scratching your nose for five minutes, what that equates to is a five-minute gap getting stuck in your head for the rest of the day. This means when someone comes up to you at work and metaphorically makes your nose itch, you don't scratch it. You just sit there and observe them. It's a nice feeling, like a subtle vibration. And if you can sit there for twenty minutes without moving, that's a twenty-minute gap you can leverage all day long.

If you get this gap in your mind, you will realise that you're so much more balanced, even if you only put a two or three-minute gap in there, it will last all day. It's the most magnificent thing.

People reference time by liquid moving through their mind and body. If your brainwave speeds slow down or speed up, that reference of time gets warped quite significantly. When you first start meditating, set a timer or two, because you'll think it was five minutes, when it was twenty. Or you'll think it was twenty minutes, and it'll only be two.

But after months, if not years, of meditation, your brain will never slow down again, and you'll be able to meditate exactly twenty minutes to the second. From the time you start meditating, your brain cycle is going to rise up and sit right on forty cycles per second, which is the ultimate speed the brain can travel, to have every single function you ever want, running at its absolute prime. It's the most bizarre phenomena.

Meditation should be practised for enough time to get the maximum enjoyment from life and not a minute more, because if you get trapped in these deep, long sits, you might be using it as a form of escapism.

The purpose of morning meditation is not reacting. If you don't react, you've created a gap that lasts all day long. But if you wake up the next day, and you don't do it again, the gap is gone. It's only there when you stick it in your head first thing in the morning.

Is there any particular method of meditation that's better than others? Is a special room or a particular kind of lighting needed?

Meditation is easy to do. There are no tricks to it. It's one of the most basic behaviours any human being can get good at.

First thing you want to do in the morning is trap a gap in your mind. You know what's easier than getting out of bed? Staying in bed. If you want to learn how to meditate, don't get out of bed. There are people who say, "I have this special meditation room with a meditation cushion and my meditation incense with my meditation music," but all of that just stands for roadblock, roadblock, roadblock. My advice is to meditate in bed, but not lying down. Once you become proficient at it, you can get your meditation room. But start in bed, because it's easier.

There are only three real principles to meditation.

▶ **Principle One: stay still**

Not scratching your nose is a metaphor for life. If you sit there for five minutes with the itchiest nose ever and don't scratch it, you've now sacrificed the animal at the altar. I'm not talking about lambs and sheep, but the hindbrain. It means telling this thing that wants to eat your nose that you're the master of it.

Once you can sacrifice the animalistic nature of your brain, you control it, so stay still.

▶ **Principle Two: breathe naturally**

If your breathing is shallow, let it be shallow. If it's heavy, let it be heavy. Don't change it. There are people who when they meditate, count their inhale for a count of five, hold it for a count of five, and then exhale for a count of five. If you're doing that, it's perfectly fine, but it's not meditating. It's counting breaths. I'm not disparaging it, because it's a great yogi practice. But again, it's breath work.

So if your goal is to meditate, don't change your breath. Because if you're doing that, you're reacting to life as opposed to allowing it to be as it is.

▶ **Principle Three: focus on the breath**

Just focus on your breath. If your mind wanders off, which is invariably going to happen, bring it back to your breath. You may even go five minutes before you realise you haven't been focusing on it.

People treat meditation aggressively. They think to themselves, *Come on, brain. Back to the breath, man. I told you what to do. What are you thinking?* Well, that's not going to help you reach a state of inner peace.

The second you realise you're not focusing on your breath, just imagine it as your best friend, and think, *Hey, best friend. Come on back to the breath. Yeah, it's okay. I know you have lots on your mind. It doesn't matter. Back to the breath, and forget about it.* Then when two seconds later it wanders off again, think, *Hey, come on back to the breath. Yeah, I know you've done it forty times already, but just come back again.*

You need to have infinite patience with bringing it back to the breath. You can't say that after ten times you're going to be really pissed off. No matter how many times it wanders off, gently bring it back.

Is there a good meditation exercise to put all of these into practice?

Yes. Here are a few things to know before you begin.

1. Sit perfectly still with your feet flat on the floor, and don't cross anything. This position is simply a better way of getting energy flow for other practices you can do later on.

If you choose to sit on the floor, cross your legs, but don't do full lotus. In the Western world, our hips and joints weren't designed for it. However, if you're easily able to, then go ahead and do it.

2.   Do whatever you want with your hands. Just don't hold a position with your arms out and fingertips touching. This means no yoga mudras, because then you have to consciously make sure your fingertips are touching, or they open up.

Try interlocking them and putting them in your lap, so that way you know they're not going to move anywhere.

3.   Focus on your breath, and breathe naturally. When your mind wanders, bring it back.

If your nostrils are clear, breathe through them. It's the way you were designed as a species. You were never, ever meant to breathe through your mouth. You're meant to eat with it. However, if your nose is blocked, then go ahead and breathe through your mouth.

If you're breathing through your nose, focus on the area in the sort of triangle around your nostrils, above your upper lip. The sensation of the breath blows across the top of your lip, adding a mouth sensation. If you're breathing through your mouth, focus on the sensation of your breath crossing your lips.

4.   Any time you get lost, gently bring it back.

Here's the meditation. It's a pretty easy process. I'm not trying to replace your practice at all, but try this technique, and note the differences. Doing your own research is the most important thing. If meditation works, it works. It doesn't matter how you do it. There are many paths to the top of the mountain, and the view is always going to be the same.

Now, meditate for as long as you can at step six. It can be five minutes, eight minutes, or longer. The better you get at this, you will need to set your alarm. When you're ready to come out of the meditation, start from step seven onwards. It's a really nice way to finish up.

1. Make sure your feet are flat on the floor, and gently close your eyes.

2. If you have to do one last little wriggle, go ahead and make that adjustment. Get it out of your system before sitting perfectly still.

3. Set the intention that you are a stone-chiselled statue. Don't move anything. Don't twitch a shoulder. Don't move a finger. Don't wriggle a toe. No matter what your body tells you it wants to do, don't move your body. Just allow yourself to meditate.

4. Let yourself breathe naturally. Focus on your breath, and observe whatever it's doing. If your breathing is shallow, let it be shallow. If it's deep, let it be deep.

5. Focus all of your awareness and attention on your breath. Observe it going in and out of your body, while not moving a single muscle. If something itches, do not scratch it. Don't be tricked. No matter what the sensation, don't move a muscle. It's time to retrain the body, so it knows you're in control, not the other way around.

6. If for any reason your mind begins to wander, gently bring it back. You are bound to be successful. You're destined to be successful. Sit still, and breathe naturally.

7. Take a nice, relaxing, deep breath, and do a full-body smile. Begin by imagining or pretending that you're beaming this incredibly vibrant smile out of the soles of your feet. The absolute biggest smile you can possibly do with your feet.

8. Allow that smile to work its way up your legs, your shins, and to your calves.

9. Smile out of your knees; a big, bright, golden smile.

10. As you smile out of your feet and knees, allow that joy to work its way up through your thighs, until you smile out of your hips.

11. Let that smile to work its way up through your abdomen, the small of your back and out of your belly.

12. As that smile works its way up, imagine smiling this warm, joyous smile out of your palms.

13. Allow that smile to work its way up your arms, until you're smiling out of your elbows.

14. Then let that smile work its way up into your shoulders, until you're smiling out of your shoulders.

15. Now your chest is opening up. Smile from the centre of your heart, out into the room. Fill the room up with warmth, joy and love from your smile.

16. Now smile out of your back. Allow it to work its way up from the soles of your feet and up through your shins, your knees, your thighs, hips, and palms. That smile works up through your chest and opens up your heart before working up into your shoulders.

17. Let that smile make its way up your neck and push through onto your face to fully express itself completely out to the world.

18. Allow your smile to travel up to the top of your head, so that every

single cell in your entire being is smiling from the top of your head to the tips of your toes, and all the way out through your fingertips.

19. With that nice big smile on your face, take a relaxing deep breath in, and as you exhale, try to extend that smile above you by reaching your arms up towards the roof, and then gently reach down towards the ground. Now slowly come back into an upright position.

20. Wiggle your fingers and toes while keeping that nice big smile all the way through your body and on your face, and gently open your eyes. Keep wiggling your toes and fingers with a big smile.

How does meditation lead to top-down management?

Paul D. MacLean refers to the neocortex, which is involved in higher functions such as sensory perception, initiation of motor commands, spatial reasoning, conscious thought and language. When you elevate into the neocortex, you do something called top-down management, which means you govern the rest of the system, whereas bottom-up management is where you're just reacting to everything that happens.

The neocortex tells the entire system what it does or doesn't do.

You can override your system. What's happening at a metaphysical or even scientific level, is that you can learn exactly how to do those processes through meditation.

Because until you start living from the top down, you do what seems natural. If you're walking down the street at three in the morning and hear a loud noise behind you, your body gets into defence mechanism. This is checkpoint one, which is your instincts. Then you turn to see what it is, which is checkpoint two, the realm of imagination. You pattern match the image and see it's cats, so you go on to checkpoint three, intelligence, and ask yourself why cats are out there.

You go through these checkpoints whenever someone or something startles you.

You're never going to be walking down the street at three in the morning, hear a loud noise and think to yourself, *Why are there cats?* It defies logic. That's why few people ever get to live top-down. It defies all of the logical programming you think you've been given.

If you can go through life doing meaningful work without anything throwing you off course, you will live true to your mission. There will be no distractions. You'll go from the neocortex, down the brainstem, and into the heart, the soul and the third eye. Now you're experiencing authentic living. That's the epitome of authenticity.

How do meditation and brainwaves relate to trauma?

Some people's brainwaves go down when meditating, instead of up. This is Delta Meditation. It happens from time to time. The reason is that after experiencing a major trauma and spending most of your time in beta mode, when you get traumatised, you spike down as low as you can go and store the trauma down there to protect yourself. Because if all your traumas in life were stored at this higher frequency, you couldn't operate.

When you first start meditating, the brain and the body say, "All right. You're meditating. You're gaining control. You've refrained from scratching your nose, and you're keeping your legs still. If you're in that level of control, we may as well start some healing now". Then it drops you down to where all of these traumas are and releases them out of the body. But it only does that once it realises you're not moving and are in control.

For the first couple of months you spend meditating, you'll actually dip down into all of these traumas, and sometimes you'll finish a meditation with quite a lot of aggression in the body. That's fine. Don't judge it. Just get on with your day. After a while of doing this, there will no more traumas left. You'll close your eyes to meditate, and go straight up to gamma. But until you clear out all the stuff at those lower brainwave frequencies, you'll always dip down when you meditate. As you clear it out, you stop concentrating on it.

What techniques do you use to achieve your goals?

I'm a big fan of falling in love with the process. People tend to fall in love with the outcome. I would also say you need to understand the power of reverse engineering. I like to get my goal into the smallest bite-sized chunks possible.

It's about breaking the goals down small enough and deliberately practicing each one, but most people sabotage their goals by making their actions too big.

Here are the steps:
1. Fall in love with the process.
2. Break it down into smaller chunks.
3. Look for habits, not goals.

A habit-oriented mindset says that if you want to write a book, forget about writing a book. Just form the habit of writing four-hundred words a day. Even if you wrote a hundred words a day, every couple of years a book would fall out of you whether you liked it or not. Habits allow you to complete a series of actions on a regular basis that delivers your goals, whether you like them or not.

What important lesson have you learned from your life experiences?

This is going to sound really clichéd. If you look back through history, at all of the different mystics and gurus in the world of transformation, most agree you have to be childlike and playful. A common phrase they use is, "Do what you love". So, if there's anything I've learned along my journey, it's to not take life too seriously.

If you're sitting around all day long, sleeping on the couch, lethargic from all of the food you're eating, you're going to constantly be drained, tired and sleepy, and won't have time to do what you love. It winds up being a catch-22. Do you find the time to do what you love before you love yourself? Or do you love yourself and then go and do what you love? I don't have the answer as to which comes first, but what I do know is that you can't have one without the other. A lot of people battling with weight issues have no energy because of a lack of self-love and self-worth.

Fundamentally, if you want to lose weight or have more energy, you need to start doing what you love. Obviously, you have to do the mindset work as well and deal with whatever shame and guilt is underneath the surface. But a great first step would be to make one list of everything you love, and another of what you do daily, and then adjust accordingly, until both lists pretty much line up with each other. Then you're good to go.

I think people need to take it easy and enjoy the ride. If you don't take yourself lightly, you're going to be heavy all of your life, so you need to lighten up a little bit. It's all a big game, and we're here to have fun and experience as much love as possible. The better you play the game, the more love you can experience, and that's kind of the reward for knowing you're playing the game correctly.

Be childlike and playful, and at all costs, make sure you do what you love. This really is the secret to elevating your energy.

To discover more about how Ben can help you *Elevate Your Energy*, simply visit www.elevatebooks.com/energy

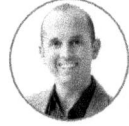

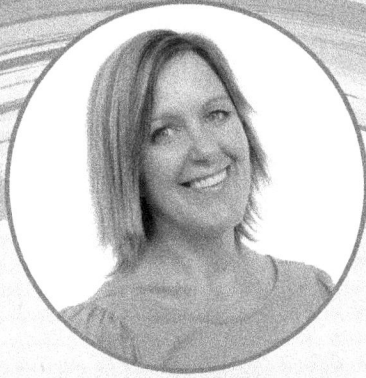

Andrea Peebles

Winning at Life

Andrea Peebles is a certified life coach, detox specialist, herbalist, personal trainer, motivational speaker, author and adventurer.

Fuelled by her father's death in 2009, Andrea left New Zealand to travel the world on a mission of adventure, and discovered that anything was possible.

Andrea has cycled through fifteen countries, run businesses as a digital nomad, raced as a professional athlete in multiple world championships and meditated with Buddhist nuns in Thai monasteries.

She's been featured on TV and in magazines, and more recently, transformed her health through fasting and detoxing.

Andrea has over twenty years of experience transforming lives. She's dedicated to helping people reach their ultimate potential and re-ignite their lives by creating a life they love.

Andrea Peebles

Winning at Life

What is the best thing that has ever happened to you, and why?

It was 2009, I had just come back from six months traveling solo overseas and moved to Christchurch to be with my fifty-years-young father, who was dying of prostate cancer. I had no job, no friends and no real purpose, other than watching his body deteriorate and waiting for him to die.

I'd broken up with my long-term partner and months earlier had a traumatic abortion. I was distraught and broken on the inside but showing a smiling face to the world. My father's large family was always present, but I was deep in loneliness. No one knew how I was really feeling. Hell, I didn't even know, being unable or unwilling to express myself or look deep within. I was brought up that way. Showing emotion seemed like a weakness. The sayings, "Don't cry over spilt milk" and "The world doesn't revolve around you", were etched deep into my psyche.

I struggled to communicate with my dad as he drifted in and out of his morphine-fuelled sleep. I desperately longed to connect and encapsulate his life experiences and wisdom from him, but often I sat in silence, feeling like a soccer ball was wedged in my mouth. And when I was alone, I cried so hard, my body convulsed as I struggled to breathe.

I found books on personal development, mindset and spiritual teachings at the library, and scrawled daily notes in my journal. I cried as I read over and over again, *Everything that happens...is the best possible thing to happen.*

Elevate Your Energy

I settled into a routine of daily exercise, meditation and yoga, and even tried fasting. I found it both a reprieve and a way into my feelings, but not knowing how to deal with them, I turned to food to suppress it all. This fuelled deep disgust with myself, so as a form of punishment, I exercised for hours. By all accounts, I was heading towards a serious disease.

One day my father, the back of his hair tufted as someone who spent his days in bed, decided to confide in me. He'd had what society would consider a great life, including a successful business, overseas holidays, a close family and a body strong enough to run marathons. But at fifty years of age, he said he wished he'd done and travelled more. He would never get the opportunity to do so.

There's something life-changing about watching someone you love have serious regrets about their life and being unable to ever fulfil them, while your capable body lives on. It pushes and pulls and ignites a flame from within you that's determined not to have the same remorse.

After witnessing my father's last laboured breath, I was motivated to get the most out of life, but I almost didn't leave. Having recently completed the infamous Coast to Coast 287km multisport race across the South Island of New Zealand, and surprising myself by placing tenth woman, my inner belief and confidence ignited just a little more. If I could do this, what else could I accomplish? But the unknown was scary, and life wasn't too bad in New Zealand...or so I told myself. Over and over again, I'd read that life begins at the end of your comfort zone. That newly ignited flame demanded more fuel. I wanted to do what I'd been taught: dare to be the brave one. So I took the leap and flew!

My father dying so young, and all of the trauma and pain I went through, was truly the best thing that happened in my life. To this day,

I'm determined not to utter those self-destroying words, "I wish I had…" I truly love my life and am dedicated to helping people transform their bodies, minds and lifestyles, so they too, can reach their potential and create a life they love.

How has adventure and travel helped you in life?

Although I'd travelled through Southeast Asia for six months in my twenties, it all up-levelled for me after watching my father have his life cut short and racing the 287km Coast to Coast. It ignited the trajectory to truly challenge my body and mind and see what else could be possible.

I've now travelled throughout the world, interweaving with different cultures and having amazing experiences. I rode my bike solo 3000km from the top of Scotland to the bottom of England, ran 130km across England, and participated in adventure races from a few hours to six-day, non-stop expedition races. The essential theme was…*sleep if you dare*.

I became a professional athlete, racing throughout Australasia. I lived out of my van in New Zealand as I trained for two world championship events and podiumed multiple adventure racing, mountain biking and trail-running events in China, Thailand, Malaysia, Australia and New Zealand.

I placed second at the Aussie Championship 24-hour Obstacle Race, my second one ever, and won my first 24-hour mountain bike race with an unsuitable bike and no specific training.

I set up my business, Re-Ignite Life in Brisbane and travelled by bike all throughout Southeast and Central Asia, Europe, Brazil, and Australia, including six months solo cycling 'the Stans'. I also completed a ten-day silent meditation retreat in the Philippines and lived with Thai Buddhist nuns while coaching as a digital nomad. I constantly harboured the belief that anything was possible and kept pushing myself to new mental and physical levels. But underneath it all, I was coming from a place of lack, doing more and more to prove myself, but never being truly satisfied. Now, I seek to enjoy the journey.

Travel and adventure have been the most challenging but incredibly rewarding experiences, transforming my life in such profound ways. Times where I thought I just couldn't continue further, and then I found it in me. The benefits are monumental. The value of immersing yourself in the challenges and beauty of life can help you understand just how capable you really are.

What are you most proud of?

While living in Brisbane, I was juggling a successful adventure training and life success studio with my athletic career. On advice from my business coach, I decided to fully pursue my athletic career and left for New Zealand to train for the World Multisport and World 24 Hour Mountain Bike (24HR MTB) championships, spaced only six days apart, because only doing only one wouldn't have been enough of a challenge!

My goal was to podium in the Multisport race, and at the eleventh hour was set to make that a reality, until I was passed on the last few kilometres of the kayak. But the 70km cycle into the finish was up, and cycling was my strongest leg. A short while into the course, I passed someone on the side of the road who I believed was my opponent.

My support crew were holding up two fingers, so I figured I was two minutes ahead. I was going to be third! I knew I had another world championship event in six days' time, so I kept my heart rate low and settled into an easy rhythm. With a feeling of elation, I crossed the finish line. That's when I was told I was fourth. I'd actually been two minutes behind. I broke down, knowing I'd had so much more in me and could have pushed myself harder. I was devastated and vowed I would never leave anything in the tank ever again.

Six days later, I lined up for the 24HR MTB, deciding after my upset to pursue the elite category. Determined to push my limits and reach my potential, after riding over twenty-four hours nonstop, I screeched across the finish line, where I fell to the ground and cried. I'd ensured another fourth placing in the world, but this time, I'd fulfilled my promise to myself. My body was broken and exhausted, but my spirit was smiling. I'd done so much more than I believed I could. I'd redeemed myself and was shocked yet again how anything was possible, as long as I stayed true to myself, kept a strong and focused mindset and had the right support.

I felt like a winner.

Why is mindset important?

Mindset is so important, because our mind is our biggest barrier to everything we want in life. When we boil everything down, we have two vibrations: love and fear. What we want, actually wants us, but our fear that comes from past trauma and pain, societal influence and conditioning, and the stories we tell us ourselves, gets in the way. We can create or destroy with our mindset alone!

When I furthered my university education into understanding mindset and human potential, and raced and trained with various athletes, I saw firsthand that what set the world-class athletes apart was their mindset. Incredibly strong athletes could crumble under pressure, but it wasn't due to lack of physical training, and being a witness to this motivated me.

I wasn't the most skilled, strongest or talented athlete by a long shot, but I always believed that ninety percent of success was through the mind, so I worked hard to strengthen it and openly believed in myself. By identifying and working in collaboration with my shadow self (the hidden parts of yourself you perceive as weak or wrong), busting my limiting beliefs and consciously flooding my mind with powerful affirmations, I created opportunities for growth and pathed my way to success beyond my wildest dreams.

My mindset and strong belief in myself have also supported me during my many solo travels all over the globe. I believe the world is a friendly and safe place, and that's exactly what I get; amazing experiences with kind people. I truly believe our outer world is a reflection of our inner one. It all starts and ends with our mindset.

What decisions have you made that caused your life to change?

Decisions form your trajectory. Yet needing to know the answer or how to get there, isn't. This is the power of belief and trusting that whatever transpires is the best thing to happen for you. It's the power of mindset and manifestation in action.

I was on my first proper solo cycling experience in England and France, and on my first day, I accidentally left my bike pump, repair kit and tools on the side of the road. After arriving in France, I scoffed at the €20 to replace them, tuned into my intuition and decided that I wouldn't need them. Of course, now, as a seasoned solo traveller, I understand that was a little too much on the optimistic side! After two and a half weeks of cycling, there wasn't one creak out of my £75 bike. Was this the power of mindset or blind luck?

In 2012, after studying to become a personal trainer, cycling 3000km solo and running 130km across England, I made the decision to live in Brisbane and open up my dream adventure and personal training studio, without having any idea how I'd make it happen or knowing anyone who lived there.

I wanted part-time work to cover expenses, but was told it was hard to get a job. I refused to believe it and was offered three out of the three jobs I applied for.

Having completed an adventure race five years earlier with only a fifty-dollar unsuitable road bike and having neither a team nor gear, I made the decision to race again. I met a man named Trevor Mullens, and when I told him about my goals, he invited me to his multimillion-dollar home. The basement was kitted with commercial gym equipment and a private garden. There was a spare bedroom I could rent while I trained and helped develop his adventure racing team, and I also ran my incredible Re-Ignite Life Studio from there. It was even better than I could've imagined!

My 'decisions' kept changing my life, including

- deciding to be on TV
- being featured in and writing magazine articles and newspapers
- training and racing with professional world-class athletes
- becoming a sponsored and professional athlete who solely lived off prize money
- living in multiple countries
- receiving last-minute invitations to sold-out overseas races
- cycling solo through multiple countries
- deciding that I would never get colds or flus again.

I was certain these were the things I would do, despite having absolutely no idea how they could happen, and every one of them did.

Do you believe having goals is important?

Here we go. I'm going to say it. I don't think they're important. Goals in many ways can be limiters and fuel our masculine energy to focus and succeed, which has benefits, of course, but challenges as well. When we become too narrowed in our goals, we can often miss the joy of the journey, and most importantly, close ourselves off to life's opportunities. How do we really know that the goal we've set for ourselves is what we need? So to me, striving for a particular goal can be counterintuitive.

I believe our power lies in setting intentions rather than goals. It's much better if you get tuned into the feeling you'll have when you get what you want, and then use that to drive the process. For example, let's say you've set a goal of spending a month in Cambodia. Now, I'd ask if traveling to Cambodia was your true objective, or if it was to experience adventure and exhilaration, feeling connection and passion, or being captivated by the mystique that motivated you. For some of you, it may absolutely be about going to a specific place and doing a specific thing, and in that case, I say to go for it. But it's worth diving into the desired feeling and checking it out.

For instance, let's say that while searching for temples to visit in Cambodia, you came upon half-price flights to Spain. Or maybe Mike, who ticks all of the boxes for your perfect match, invited you to visit him in France, another dream destination of yours...but you were still so determined to go to Cambodia, so you missed out on what you *really* wanted and needed.

I suggest you follow the desired feeling and not necessarily the desired result. Give the universe some wiggle room to bring you what you really need, not necessarily what you think you do. Have preferences for sure, but be open to the process of receiving what you want without being attached to the outcome. Work with a coach to help you remove blocks and get you into aligned vibration. This is key.

What is the best way to set and achieve your intentions?

Now, of course I'm biased, but I feel I wouldn't have achieved what I have in my life without a coach or mentor. So I say the best way is to get a coach!

Having someone support and challenge you to stretch, heal and grow further than you ever thought possible, as you realise and embody your greatest potential, is a gift I wish to bestow upon everyone.

Your viewpoints are limited to what you know, and a coach helps you identify and alchemise your blocks. They push you to get the most out of yourself and keep you focused on exactly what you want. There will always be bumps along the road. It's inevitable. You may want to give up. Hell, if you're anything like I am, as well as everyone I've worked with, fear and challenges will push and pull at you. Insecurities will creep to the surface, despite your clear intentions and a strong motivation to change. The ancient part of your brain that hasn't evolved with you, is designed to keep you safe, and change is not deemed as such. Then throw in your ego mind, unresolved pain and trauma, as well as the stress and toxins of your daily life, and you have some massive roadblocks in the way! Your motivation can waiver, but when you have someone constantly reminding and gently prodding you, while being your biggest cheerleader, you're super-charging your intention.

Working alongside a coach who lifts you up and has proven tools and strategies to help clear the blockages, can take so much pain, guessing and defeating self-sabotage out of the equation. I truly believe it's the best way to achieve everything you could ever want.

How has coaching helped you?

Back in 2014, I decided I wanted to be on TV. Due to what I believe is the power of mindset, only months later, I wound up applying to be on the ESPN series *Search4Hurt*. In the first part of the series, twelve people, six men and six women, compete to be the next *Search4Hurt* star. In the second part, the winning man and woman engage in challenging feats around Australia that push their body and mind.

I had five weeks to train for the 24-hour, non-stop audition competition against other strong athletes. At this time, I also met the inspiring powerhouse, five-time World Boxing Champion Sharon Anyos, while upskilling as a personal trainer at Max International School of Fitness. I asked her to coach me, and she not only excitedly agreed, but she took me on as her protege. I travelled over an hour one way to see her early mornings, three times a week. Her sessions were tough, but it was her conviction and unwavering belief in me that drove me to new physical and mental levels.

The standalone power of having a coach happened while I was sitting outside the *Search4Hurt* audition in my rental car. I was dressed in killer heels, a pencil skirt and makeup, feeling mortified while looking at the other athletes casually dressed in sportswear. I called Sharon in a panic, and she asked me a powerful question that became forever etched in my mind. It governs how I show up and influences how I coach my clients. That question was, "Who are you, Andrea?" This question made me think about the affirmation I'd assigned to myself at the time, which was, *I am inspirational, strong, smart, sexy, sassy and successful*. Sharon went on to say, "Are you the type of person who will stoop down to someone's else's level, or the type of person who will stand bold and proud and true to themselves? Sure, go and get changed and fit in, but what are you saying about, and to, yourself? Did you come here to stand out and show them who's the next *Search4Hurt* star or to blend in?"

My decision, thanks to Sharon, was easy. Of course I would walk in dressed to impress as planned. I would, indeed, stand true to my values and affirmations. Yet when it came time for taking action, it wasn't easy. It required lashings of what felt like faked confidence as I walked the tightrope of fear into that building while everyone stared at me.

Afterwards, looking at the video footage of all of us athletes walking together, I was pleased to see I stood out and felt immensely proud.

Being not only supported by Sharon, but fiercely challenged to stand firm in my truth, was an undeniable benefit of having her as my coach and mentor. To this day, I endeavour in my coaching to be a strong influence and bring out the best in my clients.

What else do you need to consider when setting intentions?

We ALL have fears, but these are merely thoughts, not actual danger. Many of us like to talk about what has, or could, go wrong. But this is giving energy towards what we don't want, and therefore that's what we'll get. Energy flows where your focus goes. The key is to focus strictly on our desires.

From a young age, we have other people's fears drummed into us, forming our limiting identity, and often our loved ones, without realising it, can pull down our hopes and dreams. They'll wrap it in concern or questions, which can cause us to doubt ourselves and often stop us from going towards what we want.

As children, we hear the following:

- *Watch out.*
- *Be careful.*
- *Don't slip.*
- *Don't fall.*
- *You might not make it.*

Then later on, we hear these words of concern:

- Did you know that so and so failed at what was most valuable to them? Do you want the same thing to happen to you?
- So how are you going to do this?
- Do you think you can do it?
- Do you know how hard it is?

Ahhhh! Please make them stop! Be careful who you let in on your dreams. We all have that loud voice in our heads that tells us we can't do it, we're not good enough, we might fail and we're not enough. We don't need to hear that from those who are closest to us. Dream-stealers often don't know what they're doing. You striving for more makes them uncomfortable and shows them up. They want you to stay at their level.

A captured crab, when placed in a bucket, will likely succeed in climbing out, but when there are multiple crabs, they'll grab onto each other, pulling each other down, thus preventing their escape.

If you're ready to bust out of your bucket, whether it's being overweight, weak, broke, unhealthy, bored, tired, or wanting to reach your ultimate potential in life, you absolutely can change and achieve success by making sure you have the right people surrounding you. Consider what your life would be like if these people lifted you up, congratulated your successes and got behind your dreams and ambitions, even telling you to reach higher? How much more would you have, do and become? So choose wisely the people you hang around the most, because they will affect you, whether you like it or not.

What do you think is the biggest problem people face?

Most of us are living a life that doesn't reflect our true values, hopes or dreams. With our light dimmed and our true essence hidden, we try our best to fit in and keep others happy.

We're not taught how to comprehend or properly communicate with the different masculine and feminine energies. Instead, we're focused on treating people how *we* want to be treated, rather than asking them how *they* want to be treated, and then following through.

A lot of us are disconnected from our emotions and controlled by our ego mind. We self-sabotage. Our self-talk is derogatory, and we're disconnected from our intuition/higher self and Mother Nature. Often, the thought of loving oneself is considered idealistic, egotistical, self-indulgent or flaky. Sadly, we're rarely taught or encouraged how to like, let alone love, ourselves.

We dumb down and suppress our emotions with food and drink, consumerism, social media and/or low-vibe and low-meaning activities. We're often time poor, and our heads are full of limiting beliefs that keep us small and unable to reach our potential.

Most of us are unhealthy without even knowing it. What we put in our bodies and on our skin, what we breathe in and cook with, and how we live our lives, is putting our bodies out of balance, making them congested and inflamed. And we're told these symptoms are normal. Doesn't everyone feel a little tired, become sick and get diseases, especially with age? Health professionals who are trained to treat our symptoms, tell us to take medication, which pushes our bodies further out of balance and into dis-ease. This way of dealing with our problems doesn't require us to make any lifestyle changes or manage the underlying cause of them.

We're indoctrinated with the belief that the world is a scary place, and the media perpetuates that travel is expensive, hard, and often not safe, especially as a solo woman.

Good things come to those who work hard, and work hard we do. Most of us are living to work and struggling to juggle so few holidays, while always feeling that our life isn't enough. We keep putting off what we really want to do, citing that when we have the money/time off/confidence/skills, that we will take the plunge...but that day never comes.

How are you currently making a difference in people's lives?

My business, Re-Ignite Life, offers online courses and personalised coaching that helps people become empowered and energised in their bodies, minds and lifestyle, so they can create a life they love.

My approach involves helping you identify and achieve success in your health, mindset, relationships and environment.

I have three online courses, with two designed to help you revitalise and rejuvenate your body and mind, and one focused on adventure and travel.

What experience and qualifications do you have that allows you to help people?

At sixteen, I taught aerobics and aquarobics. I later studied and worked as a gym instructor before going to university and getting a Bachelor of Health Science in Occupational Therapy and then a Post Graduate Certificate in Health.

I then worked as an occupational therapist before moving into qualitative research and strategy.

In 2012, I received a double diploma in Fitness Business and Personal Training, and completed my first life coaching and NLP certification. I set up an adventure and life success business, and then raced and travelled throughout Australasia as a professional athlete. In 2017, I trained as a yoga instructor, qualified as a detox specialist, studied herbalism and Reiki, and now coach people in their health and life goals.

How would you go about helping someone with health concerns?

When dealing with health concerns, you can do treatment with pharmaceutical medicine, which consists of chemical medication, radiation or surgery, or natural medicine, consisting of natural sources or herbs, to treat your symptoms.

Another path to take is detoxification, where I mostly play. It aims to treat the cause of the disease by removing toxicity from the body, and at the core identifies its role as your healer.

Understand that when the body has, for example, cancer, heart disease, arthritis, psoriasis or IBS, it didn't manifest these illnesses out of thin air. The body, germs or viruses, are not the enemy.

What's going on is that your body is sending you a sign that it needs attention. I'm not saying it's your fault, but once you become aware of it, it's your responsibility. So you need to focus on alkalising, cleaning and regenerating yourself back to true health.

Through my training as a detoxification specialist and herbalist, and my own journey of healing and working with many clients, I believe that the body is an incredible healing machine. True restoration, the deep regeneration of our cells, is available to us all through detoxifying our bodies, minds and environment, thus empowering us and setting ourselves free.

We can have the life and true health we desire.

What are the best ways people can find energy and heal their body?

Most people fear diseases, because they don't understand that the root cause of a majority of them is excess acidity and toxicity in the body, creating obstructions. But this can be cleansed, and genetic weakness strengthened. Any sign or symptom means the body is out of balance and not working optimally. Truly healthy bodies don't have skin issues, allergies, tumours, cravings, bloating, irritability, tiredness or brain fog, and don't regularly get injured or sick. Sure, these are quite common, but it's not normal in a balanced, healthy body.

There's no magic involved. It's a simple process of chemistry and cause and effect. Disease is a natural process that's due to an imbalance of the body and mind.

When we break it down, the body is a simple machine. It consists of two major fluids, blood and lymph, and trillions of cells. Every cell needs to be fed via the blood, and also requires excretion via the lymphatic system, to the kidneys and skin.

Cells get congested and damaged due to mistreating our bodies, which we often do without realising it. This causes impaired cellular function, obstructions in our lymphatic (waste disposal) system and even death. Our digestive waste can also back up and create obstructions and stagnation, which leads to illness symptoms setting in.

Many so-called diseases and sicknesses are nothing more than elimination efforts by the body to purge itself of toxins, dying/dead cells or waste.

Every six months or so, we do an oil change and service our car to keep the engine working properly, but when was the last time you checked on your own body?
Are you running with old or clogged-up engine oil?

In other words, you might have no idea your body is sluggish and congested, until you receive a diagnosis. Your symptoms might seem small and insignificant at first, and it's only later that you realise they add up to something far more serious.

In the same way we wouldn't take the septic tank out of the sewer when it's full, we don't want to blow up our bodies with surgery, chemo or medication when it's not working right. We just need to clean it out, so it can function optimally, and also stop putting the toxic and congesting materials into it, so it doesn't clog up again.

How can you cleanse and rejuvenate the body?

It's important to address what we put in and on our bodies. We also need to pay attention to what we think, feel, breathe and do, and the people and energy we're around. We can work in harmony with nature's laws by understanding cause and effect. Removing congestion and aiding the body to filter our cellular and digestive waste and toxins can be done through a return to our species-specific diet as frugivores, which means subsisting primarily on fruit. We can then cleanse our bodies with the electrical power and astringent properties of ripe, organic fruit, as well as the supporting and strengthening effects of herbs.

We also need to move our bodies and open the eliminative channels, such as our skin, bowels and kidneys, and stop bombing ourselves with food and drink. We can do this by incorporating fasting, releasing our trapped emotions and trauma, and viewing our body as already heathy and whole.

It's a fully holistic and simple approach to true health based on alkalising, detoxifying and energising the body.

But isn't too much fruit bad for you?

Just like petrol for your car, the proper food for your brain and body cells is glucose, which is a simple sugar you may have been told feeds cancer. It's not true. Simple sugars energise and strengthen cells, which is also essential in healing cancer. Fruits help pull mucus and toxins from the cells and enhance their vitality faster than any other food, including vegetables. Fructose is the highest energetic form of sugar. It requires no ATP or insulin, and enters the cells via diffusion, so it saves energy for the body.

It's refined sugar that's highly acidic and mucus-forming.

What's the biggest mistake people make in the area of detoxing/ trying to get healthy?

Attempting to do it all by themselves.

Now, let me start by saying that I absolutely believe in you and that you have everything you need to create change and take action. After all, you're reading this for a reason. But if you're anything like I am, and think you're motivated enough to do it yourself, I'd like to challenge you to understand why having a coach is so necessary. Can you get healthy and happy just eating clean/doing a juice fast for a few weeks, drinking more water, exercising, getting to bed early, meditating and maybe getting a new job?

Well yes, but let me share my experience with you....

I'd been vegan for a few years and eating a high fruit and high raw diet, while racing and traveling a lot as a professional athlete, so as I came crashing down, injured and burnt out, I searched for a natural way to heal myself. When I discovered detoxification, I knew I'd found the secret to rejuvenating my body. I'd been horrified seeing the gunk people had in their so-called healthy bodies. Surely I didn't have that stuff in me as well.

I thought I was pretty healthy, until I removed certain foods from my diet, and it felt like my world had collapsed. Five days into my juice fast, and I was in a frantic state, driving thirty minutes to the chip shop to gorge on hot chips washed down with cheap soda, and afterwards throwing it up with tears and snot streaming down my horrified face.

What on earth was I doing?

I wanted this so badly, yet here I was, self-sabotaging and destroying myself.

I was immersed stress-free in nature, surrounded by likeminded people, had daily, sometimes multiple, meditation sits, yoga sessions and forest walks, and yet on the inside I was screaming.

Removing food and drink left me vulnerable and exposed, my suppressed emotions now naked, raw and demanding attention. I was also oblivious to a heavy parasite and fungal infestation in my body, which fed my out-of-control cravings and binges. I then drowned in guilt and disgust, feeling so helpless and alone. I couldn't understand what was going on or how to pull myself out of it, even with my tools as a certified life coach and what I'd learned in my training to become a detox specialist and herbalist. I struggled alone, hiding in shame. I felt I should've been able to sort myself out. It was a turbulent time.

Detoxification isn't only a physical experience, but a mental, emotional, spiritual and environmental one. It took me many years of huge peaks and troughs, restriction and binging, trying and failing, and so much self-directed hate that could have been avoided on my detoxification journey.

It sure doesn't need to be that way. In fact, I believe getting healthy is actually a fun and simple experience! If only I'd had a coach who could help me navigate my healing journey as we worked through my trapped emotions, pain, fears and cravings, while giving practical support, which is what I do now for others.

I can't recommend enough investing in life-changing support by a qualified and experienced coach you vibe with, trust and who fully understands what's going on.

What is the best tip you could give someone?

Take responsibility for your life. Dream big. Figure out what you really want and who you are, and then work with someone to help you align with it. Remove limiting beliefs and blocked emotions, and reframe traumatic and painful experiences. Set high standards for yourself. Stop living a life that's less than you're capable of. Be the star in your own show. Find someone who will support and challenge you and take action. Start being that person who has what you want right now. This is key, because you need to be it before you see it. Relax into life, flow with what comes up and trust that everything happening is for your highest good. Learn from your failures, knowing that failure is feedback, and rejection is only redirection.

Get out and experience life in all its vibrant messiness. Travel far and wide to see the incredible beauty of the world and its people. Plan adventures that challenge, push and pull you to new levels, and show you what you're made of. Immerse yourself in nature. Create a life you passionately love, and know that you have the power and potential to achieve whatever you want, with your ultimate partner and your ideal tribe. Learn how to navigate the masculine and feminine dance. Buckle in, and enjoy the magic ride.

And specifically, take time to cleanse and strengthen your body. Detoxify it physically, mentally, emotionally and environmentally, and understand that a lifetime of trauma, toxins and unhealthy habits got you here. You're fighting against generations of unhealthy living, so it will take more than a few weeks to do this. Likely years. There's no quick fix or hack, and if you find one, it's at most fleeting and likely harsh. True healing happens when you get to the root cause and address it lovingly, in harmony with nature's laws, and allow the body to do the work.

You don't need easy you're built of strong stuff. Challenges uncover who you truly are. Make a decision that you are worthy and deserving to look, feel and have vibrant, true health and long-lasting energy. And if at all possible, work with a coach to unblock any resistance that comes up.

Make a commitment to your health. Challenge yourself to make it a priority. Vibrant health is the cornerstone of a vibrant life. It's so worth it. You're so worth it.

To discover more about how Andrea can help you *Elevate Your Energy*, simply visit www.elevatebooks.com/energy

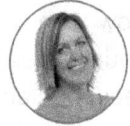

Elise Peck

The Law on Love

Elise Peck is a love, relationship and intimacy coach who helps people uncover their authentic, attractive energy.

Elise's background includes careers as a lawyer, dancer and entrepreneur. In time, her own longing for deep authentic love, connection and intimacy, took her on a journey of discovery to crack the code of how people become a magnet for the love they desire.

Elise helps her clients transform loneliness and longing, into deep connection. She helps her clients to heal and transcend addictive toxic relationship cycles, and to attract the love they desire. With renewed passion and energy, her clients experience a deep sense of self-love and self-worth, attract more abundance, finally feel well in their body and live a life in alignment with who they really are.

Elise is a highly effective Relationship Coach, passionate about her clients and their results.

Elise Peck

The Law on Love

What is your biggest life lesson?

My biggest life lesson is that the magic happens on the other side of surrender.

That moment when you finally 'let go' is where the juice is.

When you drop into acceptance of the moment, and all resistance falls away, that's when your desires come streaming towards you (or something even better).

From my experience, unmedicated childbirth was the ultimate real-time, tangible experience of this life lesson. When the birthing experience reaches the 'transition' phase, right before you're on the edge of the breakthrough, and you're closer than ever to attaining what you're seeking, anxiety and fear will peak. It all feels like too much, so you look for the exit button.

But in childbirth, once you've reached the 'transition' phase, there is no exit button. It's too late to get pain medication at this point, even if you wanted it, and there's nothing left to do in that moment but surrender. The more you resist and spiral into the fear, the more you stall meeting your child.

When you let nature take its course and work its way through you, you'll be able to dive into the abyss. By opening yourself up to the fear and accepting the pain and challenges that arise, you can reframe the experience as something that's serving you, and the outcome you're seeking happens a lot quicker. In this case, you'll be able to enjoy that newborn in your arms.

Elevate Your Energy

What does love mean to you?

Essentially, I believe there are two opposing forces in life: love and fear.

The relationship you have with yourself dictates the one you have with life and others. So I really like to bring the focus to what it means to love, trust, appreciate and accept yourself, which feels like listening to your intuition and following your curiosity without judgement, shame, guilt, embarrassment or fear.

On the other hand, not loving yourself means you're moving the way fear moves you.

I also believe that we can only truly learn to love ourselves through relating to others.

We need relationships to mirror back our edges and shine a light on the parts we've hidden from ourselves.

True love comes about when we simultaneously work on loving and accepting ourselves, in conjunction with loving and accepting others.

Our intimate relationships, our relationship with our children and our relationship with ourselves, combine to create the ultimate self-development pathways to understanding unconditional love, if we approach them with that intent.

If you were speaking to your younger self, what advice would you give?

Find the tools to neutralise your trapped emotions, transcend your limiting beliefs and heal your attachment wounds.

In addition, it's SO important to trust and follow your intuition, which is the quiet, calm voice inside. I like to call it "following your curiosity", and I've found this to be the key to your creativity, living your truth and being in flow with life. Sometimes people will tell you to "listen to your gut", but I've found this can often lead you off your path. The reason is that fear often shows up as a gut feeling. So, when you have a chaotic, anxious or tight feeling, pause, dive into it and extract the wisdom, but resist taking any action from that place. The best decisions come from a calm mind.

Please take your time fully opening to people, and be wary of any relationship that has an urgent or fast feeling about it. Amazing, healthy, fulfilling relationships, and amazing things in general, take time.

What would you like your legacy to be?

I would love my legacy to be that I helped people heal from their childhood wounds, so they could return to love and be more loving role models for the next generation.

I want to be remembered for guiding people back to the lost wisdom of the masculine and feminine dance, so they once again came alive and found the joy, spark, excitement and zest for their life. I would love my legacy to be that I helped create incredible, healing, intimate relationships, alive with the powerful force of sexual energy, and how the healthy union of masculine and feminine energies can be used to create their ultimate vision for life and love.

Have you had any aha moments that changed everything for you?

A *major* aha for me was realising I could totally change my life experience by igniting, uncovering and nurturing my authentic, attractive, feminine self and become energetically attractive to the love I desired.

Learning about polarity in relationships, and how to actually create chemistry and desire in intimate relationships, changed everything. I was absolutely shocked to observe just how differently my husband related to me when I changed my polarity. I couldn't believe I had that untapped power sitting inside of me the whole time.

What decisions have made a difference in your life?

A massive decision I made that changed my life was when I dedicated an entire year to healing my toxic cycles, up-leveling my physical self and solving why things weren't going how I desired. I spent time diving into emotional pain and discovering the tools to neutralise and transcend those cycles.

What's the best thing that has ever happened to you, and why?

Discovering how to heal from childhood attachment wounds to create a secure attachment style for myself. Prior to my healing journey, I didn't trust anyone. At my lowest point, I felt the world was an unsafe place, and people were constantly 'having a go' at me. I couldn't accept support from anyone other than my husband. I had the attitude of "if it is to be, it's up to me", and I was fiercely independent.

Consequently, I spent well over three years parenting 24/7 without a break. Even though my husband says he's always loved me deeply and consistently, I couldn't actually trust or feel the depth of his love, until I healed my many triggers and inner wounds. I had a constant vigilance, which was exhausting and meant I was always on high alert. It made me jumpy, anxious, worried and defensive. I was high-strung. My emotions were erratic, amplified and overwhelming.

My mind was consistently noisy, running over past hurts or trying to figure out the precise meaning of past conversations and if a person was purposely trying to hurt me. It was like my mind kept re-traumatising me.

Since healing, my emotions are so much calmer, my mind more peaceful and clearer, and I can witness my emotions and thoughts with awareness. I now consciously choose my response, rather than unconsciously reacting or suppressing it. As my mind is free from inner turmoil, it has a lot of time for creation, and my creativity has exploded. I attribute this partly to my cultivation of sexual energy, to living a life in alignment, and to neutralising past traumas.

What's your big WHY?

I want to help adults who've felt scared, traumatised, powerless or damaged in the past. I want to see them heal and become thriving, functioning adults who enjoy fulfilling, healthy and psychologically safe adult relationships.

My goal is to relieve people of the terrible loneliness and powerlessness that results from feeling like they can't get the love they desire in life.

My Why stems from feeling so powerless and lonely before I turned inward and found the power inside of me. It's a really challenging place to be, where you're stuck in the longing for deep connection, belonging and love.

I found the answers, and frankly, it would feel selfish of me if I didn't pass on this empowering, life-changing wisdom to others.

What do you think is your life purpose?

Empowering people to live their authentic truth.

What do you believe you've been put on the planet to do?

To support people in their return to love, which includes acceptance of their authentic self. I want to teach them how to love themselves, connect deeply with others and have a life of abundant, vital energy, so their spark for life is reignited.

How are you currently making a difference in people's lives?

I love working with clients one-on-one as a relationship coach, assisting them in attaining the connection and intimacy they desire. I receive frequent messages from women giggling with joy about the men now pursuing them. They're often surprised to find way more abundance flowing into their life in the way of opportunities, money, clients, ideas, creativity, training and unexpected gifts.

What I notice the most, is that there's a total, undeniable energetic shift. I'm often wowed by how different they sound.

Both the men and women I've worked with find themselves getting *way* more romantic attention and interest while working with me. They're excited about life and feel more attractive. It's really quite fun and often hilarious listening to their stories.

I'm also passionate about helping clients transcend toxic relationship cycles. Many of them come to me feeling addicted to people they know aren't a healthy match. I empower clients to only accept and invest in relationships that reflect their value and worth. Once they heal the parts of themselves that are attracted to unhealthy dynamics, and learn to let go of them, it creates space to allow in healthy love. They're amazed and so appreciative of just how well they're treated in healthier relationships.

What are you passionate about?

Helping people understand how to keep the attraction, passion and energy in their relationships and love life long-term, so they feel safe, connected, and loved. They heal the inner wounds keeping them stuck in loneliness and fear, and enter into relationships that reflect their value and worth. I also love helping clients repair their current relationships and learn to love their life and live their truth, so they can step into their power.

What's the best way to help them with this problem?

They need to get an excellent and passionate coach. With me by your side, we'll work together to overcome your fears and the constant sabotage and unhealthy cycles that are keeping you trapped in your unfulfilling reality.

What's the biggest mistake people make in the area of intimate relationships?

The biggest mistake people make is not realising they have the power to change their circumstances. They get caught up in what the other person is or isn't doing, or they're focused on what's showing up externally in their life. Instead, they need to go within and work on their own stuff, so they can awaken their power to attract the love they desire.

The basic foundations (secure base) of a relationship are definitely crucial, but polarity is what keeps relationships alive.

Relationships are like plants. They need to be watered and nourished, and the weeds need to be tended to and pulled out.

For ongoing fulfillment in romantic relationships, it's crucial to understand how to nurture yourself into your own masculine or feminine pole, while supporting your partner more into their opposing one.

For example, the masculine should be aware that the feminine needs to feel seen, cared for, respected and understood in order to open up, and the feminine should be aware that the masculine needs to feel appreciated, accepted, needed and also challenged (to a certain degree). Once you consciously make time to engage with your partner in a way that nurtures their polarity, it allows an attractive energy to flow between you, enlivening the relationship and your life.

How did you become interested in helping people improve their intimate relationship?

Twelve years into my relationship with my husband, and after two children, I felt an intense loneliness and pain.

I longed to feel desired. I wanted greater intimacy and to have that spark of chemistry be more present in our relationship. I craved the feeling of attractive masculine energy desiring me and pursuing me.

What I didn't realise at the time, was that I was actually overabundant in my masculine energy, which energetically repelled my husband's. I didn't understand that the flame of my attractive feminine energy was smothered and needed to be uncovered and reignited.

The pain of wanting more intimacy, and desiring to feel desired, drove me into a deep discovery of uncovering how people attract the love they want into their life. It absolutely blew my mind that by implementing the many tools and techniques I'd uncovered, and returning to my authentic feminine energy core, the world seemed to shift around me. Not only did my husband start charging towards me with total desire, but I was more attractive to life in general. I became a magnet for love and abundance.

As my energy shifted, so did my husband's. His newly activated attraction for me and my feminine energy, drove him to also seek answers about how we could up-level the relationship, so I could feel all the love I desired. Ultimately, my quest to discover how to get the love I wanted, became an incredible healing journey for both of us. Now I'm passionate about showing everyone how they can do the same.

What are your most inspiring client stories?

- I have a client who became inundated with male attention not long after she began working with me. Her ideal man then turned up. She often sends me screen grabs of the beautiful messages he sends her. He shows up consistently and reliably and adores her. She's SO happy she was able to move on from her previous partner. This client is now absolutely GLOWING as a total goddess. The physical difference from when she first began working with me until now, is astounding.

- A client messaged me within 1 week of her first session with me exclaiming it was "hailing men", and within 3 weeks met a beautiful partner that she now has a fulfilling, highly orgasmic relationship with, beyond anything she'd previously experienced.

- A client came to me with an intimacy issue he'd struggled with for decades, and after just one session, all symptomology of the issue vanished.

- A client came to me after working with multiple coaches (including highly experienced, award-winning, high-ticket coaches), because he'd been stuck mourning a relationship that had ended thirty years previous. Within three sessions, this inner wound that had dominated his life was now released.

- A client came to me with fears around being seen and taking action on his mission in life, both of which are connected to masculine energy. Within three sessions, he was taking massive action, putting himself out on social media and diving into his mission.

- A client came to me feeling like she couldn't do anything in life if she didn't have a partner. She was even fearful of leaving her apartment on her own. She had a massive fear of being on her own, and consequently had been involved in a string of unhealthy, abusive relationships.

After our first call, she was leaving her apartment and going out for walks in the sunshine. Within two calls, she'd reawakened a forgotten passion. She was having fun, laughing, playing, and making huge strides to disentangle from a toxic relationship.

Do you have an approach to your coaching?

For women, I deliver my signature 5-step system, Glo-Flo: The most Powerful Program for Igniting Your Attractive Feminine Energy.

This system, delivered via one-on-one coaching, together with an accompanying online video program, layers women through all of the transformative steps required to attract the love they desire into their life:

Step One: Vision of Love

We go through tools and processes to get clear on what you truly, authentically want, why it's important to you and what's been preventing that vision to date.

This step is crucial to attracting a healthy relationship that's authentic to you. Often a huge mistake women make is that they attach to one specific man at all costs, and in the process, often abandon and deny what they truly want.

Getting clear on your vision allows you to be more invested in your relationship vision than in a particular person, and this gives you a more balanced approach to getting the love you want. It allows you to show up magnetic rather than needy.

Step Two: Align with Love

We get you authentically, energetically, consciously and unconsciously aligned with the love you really want. This involves processes to remove the resistance that's currently blocking healthy love and connection from manifesting in your life.

We help you identify where fear, inner conflicts and trapped emotions are preventing you from stepping into alignment with what you want, and uncover what you value, to ensure you're living an inspired life. This step also involves processes to activate the resource centres in your mind, which will then cause you to take actions that are aligned towards your vision.

Step Three: Open Your Heart

In this step, we take a deeper dive into removing the resistance that's getting in the way of you living in flow with life. Attractive feminine energy is open and receptive to love and new experiences. It's one thing to be inspired, love your life and be in your glow, but it's another to allow other people and love in.

Here we step through some powerful tools to deal with past events, limiting beliefs and fear that are closing your heart off to love, support and connection. Until you can trust in your ability to have your own back, hold your boundaries, speak your truth and make decisions from inner inspiration, you will have a hard time trusting others. Keeping your heart open is the only way you can receive all the love available to you.

Step Four: Love Yourself

In this step, we really look at healing and nurturing your own relationship with yourself. It's about owning and loving ALL parts of your body. You'll learn a powerful, sacred sexuality practise that connects you with yourself, cultivates your sexual energy and taps into incredible brain waves that allow your creativity and intuition to be turned on and flow out.

This is the most powerful step to igniting your attractive feminine energy. It's a real game-changer if you embrace and dive into the process. Your entire energy shifts, and masculine energy becomes waaaaay more drawn to you. You'll step into your power and feel a deep respect and honour for your body.

After this step, you're unlikely to accept any future situations that don't honour and respect your sacred temple. It's a coming home to yourself and builds an incredible amount of self-love, self-worth and self-value. There's a bonus lesson in here on how to orgasm on command, with no touch, if that's something you desire to learn more about, since sexual energy is creative life force energy.

Step Five: Love Others

This step is crucial. We delve into your relationships and look at how to create secure attachments.

It lays out the tools, strategies and blueprint for how healthy relationships function, how to alchemise conflict into connection and how to keep the chemistry and spark alive in relationships...forever!

You'll learn actual, tangible strategies for how to dance the masculine and feminine dance in a way that keeps the chemistry, desire and passion *alive*. There's also a masterclass on how to have conscious, multi-orgasmic sex, AKA the kind that connects you more deeply with your partner and is a true reflection of love and authentic intimacy. It's the sex education we all ought to have had.

In addition, sprinkled throughout the entire course, are extremely potent and dynamic health hacks to have you totally glowing from inside out. I'm also a certified integrative health practitioner who knows a great deal about body transformation. In fact, I also help clients get the body they desire. It's so much easier to feel steady in our mind, and love ourselves, when we feel vital and comfortable in our own skin.

These health hacks could be an entire standalone course. This information isn't just world class, it's *the* health knowledge used by the elite.

I don't hold anything back in this online course. It truly includes everything you need to ignite your Attractive Feminine Energy, and the results clients experience are mind blowing.

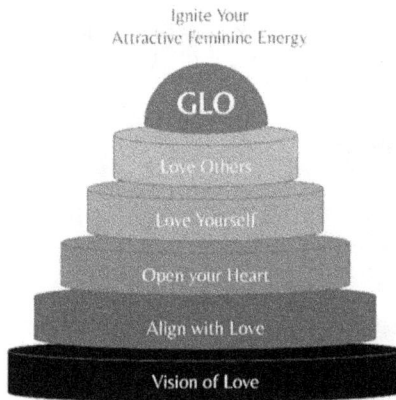

Ignite Your
Attractive Feminine Energy

GLO
Love Others
Love Yourself
Open your Heart
Align with Love
Vision of Love

For men, I have a one-on-one coaching program, Unleash Your Masculine Power, that allows you to create the love and life you desire.

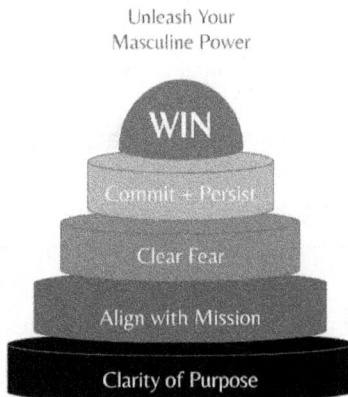

Unleash Your
Masculine Power

WIN
Commit + Persist
Clear Fear
Align with Mission
Clarity of Purpose

Step One: Clarity of Purpose

The key element of high-value, embodied masculine energy, is commitment to your mission in life. This energy of living in alignment and pursuit of your authentic purpose, makes you attractive to high-value feminine energy, and builds your self-worth, value and passion for life. It helps you develop the grit, stamina, commitment, persistence and delayed gratification required for an incredible and rewarding love and sex life. You'll feel alive and whole within yourself, so that your energy is far more attractive, and your advances towards feminine energy will be met with more interest.

The more you value yourself, the more you will only permit a relationship that reflects what you want. Before you can align with, fearlessly move toward and commit to your purpose, you must first know what it actually is. So this is the first step in your pathway. Together, we go through the tools and processes to uncover what you value and how you ought to be prioritising your time. We also use this same process to get clarity on what kind of relationship you want.

Clarity around your purpose and what you desire in life and in a relationship, also requires a level of self-awareness and depth of presence.

Step Two: Align with Mission

In this step, we identify where you have some inner conflicts, self-sabotage cycles and limiting beliefs that are preventing you from pursuing both your mission and the women you're interested in.

We'll work together to get you aligned and inspired from within. We help you identify what feelings are most important to you in life and motivate you to take new and different actions toward your mission and getting your ideal woman. If you don't clear out the confusion, self-sabotage and attachment to old programs and ways of being, you'll stay inside your comfort zone, which will prevent you from yielding new, desirable outcomes.

Step Three: Clear Fear

Sometimes we know what we want, and we feel really motivated to go after it, and then crippling fear stops us! This can look like the fear of rejection, fear of being seen and fear of failure or change. So in this step, we dive into tools that will clear the doubt around running towards your career and relationship goals.

Step Four: Commit + Persist

For both success with your mission in life and in a relationship with a high-value feminine energy, a lot of grit, commitment and persistence is required. The masculine is the penetrative, goal-oriented force in the world who must focus on what he wants. This energy is highly attractive to the feminine, who's the receptive energy. It allows for incredible chemistry and intimacy in your relationship, in and out of the bedroom.

For a woman's body to be open and orgasmic, a lot of trial and error is required from the masculine. The feminine also has many waves of emotions and is ever-changing. The masculine should aim to be the grounding lighthouse in the storm of these waves, and this requires the ability to persist without giving up.

This is also reflected in your career. The alpha male is the one with staying power, the one who's committed until he wins, or the goal is attained.

At this stage, we strategise ways to handle the challenges in both business and relationships, and use the tools and processes to create a new cycle of stoic tenacity, where previously quitting was the habitual action. We delve into the masculine/feminine dance more and discuss how to handle the challenges inherent in meeting what the feminine really needs. We help you figure out how to remain a steady presence and ensure you're nurturing your masculine energy, while also supporting her feminine energy.

All of this leads to you WIN-ing in your career (your mission), in your relationship and in life.

For those men who are interested, I also offer health coaching along this pathway as required, to support you in feeling physically comfortable and confident. I help you have a relationship with food that reflects self-love, self-respect and self-value. The feedback I've received is that this element of my coaching alone is 'priceless'.

What courses have you taken that enabled you to get started or build your business?

* Certified Results Coach
* Bachelor of Law (Honours)/Bachelor of Commerce
* Certified Integrative Health Practitioner (Health Coach)

What's the best way people can achieve a great life-work balance?

Get clear on your ultimate vision of life and what you value most. Update this as you evolve, prioritise it daily and take inspired action towards it. Understand what your core driving wound is, which I've also seen referred to as your 'mother wound' or 'highest shadow value'. Your core driving wound is basically your biggest trigger, the thing that gets a major emotional reaction from you.

In relationships, this often shows up as a 'core scene' fight, which is another way of saying it's the theme behind an argument that occurs over and over again.

Are you most triggered when you have a sense of loss of control or abandonment? How about when you feel engulfed, ignored or invalidated? Awareness of your relationship patterns, greatest inner voids (unmet needs in childhood), and strongest triggers, is key. If you don't figure out what your core driving wound is, it can totally derail you in life and in love. It's imperative that you learn what drives you and which needs are unmet, so you can fulfil them in healthy ways and turn that wound into gold. You can actually find your worth in your deepest wound, and use it as fuel for your business and life goals. Your wounds hold the gold.

How did you decide on the name and logo for your business?

I allowed inspiration to flow through me and stayed open to suggestions. Initially, I was going to call the feminine program simply GLOW, but when I was creating the program, the teacher in charge of our training, Benjamin J Harvey, happened to reference mothers getting back 'in flow' with life, and that inspired me to make the name GLO-FLO.

As for the logo, it unexpectedly fell into my lap, as things often do when you're in flow. I had an incredible brand stylist, Jaypee Toledo, create a style look-book for my brand image ahead of a photoshoot, and he spontaneously decided to also throw together a logo and included it in the brief. I loved it, so that became my logo.

Why is mindset important?

When you master your mindset, you've mastered your life.

Your beliefs create your actions, your repeated actions become your habits, your habits become who you are and who you are determines your life experiences.

How does someone keep inspired on a daily basis?

Prioritise your highest values daily. By doing this, inspiration from within picks you up and pulls you towards your goals, because it feels aligned and fun. Live a life that reflects who you are and what you authentically enjoy, and inspired action will just be your way of existing and doing life.

On the hard days, when you have commitments, but you're just not in the mood, think back on your Why. As in, why you started, why you made this commitment in the first place and why you do what you do. When the Why is accurate and true to you, you'll find an endless source of energy and inspiration. Taking care of your health and wellbeing makes you feel good in your body, have better energy and show up more inspired, too. Also, having enough downtime, play time and meditation, as well as time for cultivating sexual energy, allows inspiration to endlessly flow through you.

Tap into what you value and what your core driving wound is. Then link up the ascertainment of your goals to feeding it and the things you value most. You'll soon become addicted to the tasks that take you to your desires. Once you realise that your goals meet your deepest needs and values, you'll feel totally drawn to them.

What are the common barriers people run into?

Resistance. Everything you want is on the other side of it.

Resistance can be the fear that shows up as
1. internal mind chatter, telling you all the reasons why you can't.
2. trapped emotions, creating images in your mind that scare you away from your dream.
3. internal conflicts, that cause you to remain stuck in analysis paralysis.

Basically, the fear of leaving our comfort zone and going into the unknown is the major barrier. Our mind resists change and sees the unfamiliar as unsafe. If we can't overcome the fear of the unknown and dive into aligned risks, we stay stuck in our comfort zone.

What mindset do you believe is needed, in order to create a great life?

You need to believe that everything is always working out for you, that there's opportunity and wisdom in every experience and that you have the power to achieve anything you set your mind to.

You also need to believe that you're lovable, whole and complete, right now, and have a mindset of self-inquiry and self-awareness. You need to believe that you have incredible resilience and can handle whatever comes your way, while also maintaining a curious and open mind that seeks to continually expand and grow.

What do you believe holds most people back from achieving the lifestyle they desire?

Fear of moving outside their comfort zone and not having the tools to transcend their fears or to realise their comfort zone is actually more dangerous than growing.

Does visualisation work?

Done correctly, yes. Here's a great way to get the best results:
- Playfully hold the vision.
- Feel the feelings of living in that outcome, and trust that it's inevitable.
- Go about living your life with the energy of knowing that all that you visualise is making its way to you, and then let go of needing to see the evidence right away. Instead, try living in the state or feeling as if it's already happened.

If visualisation creates an awareness of what you don't currently have, and you end up feeling a void, then it won't work. In this case, stop visualising certain outcomes, and instead spend time simply feeling the feelings. Start noticing all of the abundance already in your life and appreciate everything, so you resonate at the vibration of abundance.

In essence, it all depends on how you relate to the visualisation and the energetic space you're in when you're doing it.

Do you have a coach or mentor, or someone who motivates you?

Yes. I have had many, many mentors.

I have a coach I really enjoy working with at the moment. She helps me to expand my worldview outside the bubble I exist in, and have a broader perspective. She allows me to realise just how much opportunity is out there. She believes in me and helps me realise my true potential. It's wonderful to have someone I trust in my corner supporting and believing in me. This feeling of support and trust also helps nurture my attractive feminine energy, which is fuelled when you feel cared for.

I have an incredible, absolute genius of a health coach. I actually ended up studying with him, and I now pass on his golden wisdom to my clients, with phenomenal results.

I've learned from a vast array of relationship coaches, psychologists, business mentors and experts, and integrate all of their wisdom, together with my personal experience with myself and my clients, into my own unique offering.

How do they make a difference to your success?

No successful person has got there on their own. It's invaluable to learn from people further down the pathway, who've achieved the results you seek.

Having a coach gives you an objective view. Often when you're so 'in' your life, you can't see it with the clarity of someone else looking in. It's also nice to have a safe space to process and move through things.

Is meditation or mindfulness something everyone should practise?

Yes. It ought to be a way of existing. You can bring mindfulness into everything you do. Having a meditation practice allows you to have far more management over how you respond to life. It gives you time to choose your response, instead of unconsciously reacting. This is priceless in relationships, where you can frequently get triggered. There's so much power in having a clear and calm enough mind to be the witness of your circumstances, and from that place choose an appropriate response. It's totally life-changing. It helps you hear your intuition and make aligned decisions.

What's your simple formula for health?

- ▶ Walk more (at least thirty minutes every day, ideally first thing in the morning before breakfast).
- ▶ Get out and enjoy the sunshine and nature.
- ▶ Master your mind.
- ▶ Do meditation.
- ▶ Have five to seven cups of vegetables every day. You can blend them up to make them easier to digest/decrease stress on the digestive system.
- ▶ Fast overnight for at least 12 hrs (ideally 6.30pm- 6.30am).
- ▶ Move to three meals per day.
- ▶ Only have liquid before lunch (the best breakfast is a smoothie).
- ▶ Limit any junk food to just one meal per week.
- ▶ PLAY.
- ▶ Laugh.
- ▶ Have fun.

Do you recommend any spiritual practices to keep your clients at their peak?

Yes. Ensure sexual energy is flowing through you and not leaking out or being left dormant. For females, work towards maintaining a sexual simmer alive in your body as much as possible. I work with clients to empower them to achieve this.

Why do you think so many people are overwhelmed and unhappy with life?

They're living a life based on external validation rather than internal inspiration. People also don't know how to counterbalance the intense mental chatter and clutter.

Why is rest and relaxation important?

This is when we heal and repair. It's also very often when creativity flows in. The best ideas happen when you're relaxed and feeling good. It also allows your hormones to stay in balance.

It's important to not burn out and have your creative juices dry up. This is in terms of your relationships as well, because some of the best bonding moments come when you're relaxing together.

People who are high-strung are going to have a hard time regulating their emotions and making clear, calm decisions. Also, intuition and curiosity whisper to us most clearly, the more relaxed we are. Listening to this quiet knowing inside is the key to living in abundance and a flow state, which brings alignment and life fulfilment.

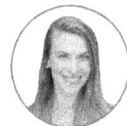

To discover more about how Elise can help you *Elevate Your Energy*, simply visit www.elevatebooks.com/energy

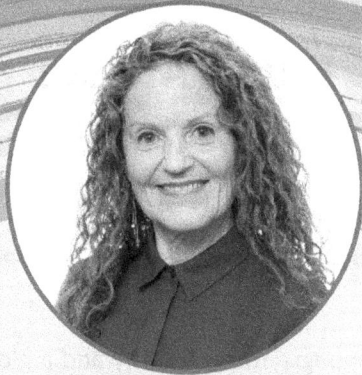

Karen Austen

The Vibe of Vitality

Karen Austen is an international speaker, bestselling author, facilitator, coach and mentor, who has a deep interest in human potential and communication.

An abrupt end to a twenty-five-year career in criminal justice changed her life drastically. After being told she'd never work again, Karen embarked on a decade-long journey of self-discovery to prove them wrong.

Through studying with masters in the field of mind-body medicine, she discovered the keys to vitality, love and abundance, and has dedicated herself to sharing them with the world.

Her approach to serving her clients revolves around her deep understanding of scientific and spiritual principles. Her mission is to let people know that the past does not have to equal the future, and thriving is possible.

Karen Austen

The Vibe of Vitality

If you were speaking to your younger self, what advice would you give?

You're more than enough. You're worthy and a glorious, magnificent creator of life and love. The world is a playground in which you can create anything you desire when you're aligned with, and connected to, who and what you really are.

Earth is a planet of embodiment, and there are some laws of nature you must be aware of in order to have the ride of your life. Discovering your essential rhythm, and becoming fluent in the languages of your body, being and nervous system, provides a powerful advantage.

You will have a body that experiences everything from pleasure to pain. These sensations are transitory, so don't hold onto them or grasp for them. Allow them to come and go.

Your body will be the physical representation of your unconscious mind. Allow it to be at its highest vibration as a vehicle for vitality, vibrancy, love and full-soul expression.

You will have a mind with higher mental faculties and a capacity to connect with a universal consciousness. These faculties are so powerful, they will create anything you feed with emotion.

You will have emotions. They are a powerful fuel and generate movement towards protection or connection. You will need someone to help you regulate them, so they don't gallop away like wild horses in any direction, taking your balance with them.

And most importantly, have fun!

What's your biggest life lesson?

I learned that I'm not loved or loveable, but that I am Love. It's who and what I am. And I am enough.

For decades, I treated my body without mercy, pushing myself to the edge by doing more than my share in every work and social environment. I was the go-to person to fix any problem, so I wouldn't feel the shame of "I am not enough". I created myself as the overachiever pleaser, in order to feel wanted and needed. All of this was at the expense of my energy, body, mind and emotional world.

My journey back to wellbeing and vitality wasn't one big 'aha' moment. It was a painstaking dance forward and backward that took years. I'd hit rock-bottom on every level of life, finances, relationships, identity, success, health and vitality. It was one step after another returning to the world of the living through every aspect of my mental, emotional, physical and spiritual being. Every part of me needed to release the limitation story in order to build a foundation of vitality, vibrancy and energy.

It wasn't until I healed at the level of my nervous system and being spiritually aligned with the higher aspects of myself, that real wellbeing was available to me. Before I regulated my nervous system, I was imprisoned in a world of post-traumatic stress, depression, anxiety, exhaustion and burnout that would dictate everything I said and did.

I also learned the highest purpose of

- the physical body, to hold the greatest level of presence (soul/spirit/self).
- the mental body, to focus will and attention on intentions.
- the emotional body, to fuel intention/vision with movement and momentum.

What was the one thing that when you got it, everything else fell into place?

Healing at the level of my autonomic nervous system (ANS), brought me alignment, connection and foundation. It returned my balance and equilibrium by moving me out of stuck survival protection modes.

Could you explain more about the autonomic nervous system?

Your nervous system runs the show!

The ANS maintains your body's internal environment and is also involved in controlling and maintaining your
* digestion
* metabolism
* urination
* defecation
* blood pressure
* sexual response
* body temperature
* heartbeat
* breathing rate
* fluid balance.

In simple terms, there are two main parts of the autonomic nervous system that are important for you to know about:

▶ **The sympathetic**
  Located near the thoracic and lumbar regions in the spinal cord, its primary function is to mobilise the body for action, and where it perceives danger, stimulate the body's fight-or-flight responses.

▶ **The parasympathetic**
  Located between the spinal cord and the medulla, it primarily stimulates the body's 'rest-and-digest', 'feed-and-breed' and social

engagement responses, as well as the survival-immobilisation-freeze response.

Survival mobilisation happens without your conscious control and instantly causes hormonal and physiological changes that allow you to act quickly. It's been part of evolution, from marine life to reptiles, and then to mammals, over hundreds of millions of years.

The freeze response (immobility) is our most ancient and highest defence mechanism. Many victims of rape have been challenged because they didn't fight back. Consider that their nervous system assessed the highest level of defence (freeze) was needed in order to keep them alive.

Have you ever witnessed or experienced something truly horrible, like an accident of some kind? Do you fixate on what you see and go numb, not feeling anything at all, even though you think you should? This is your nervous system protecting you, as it's too much to process all the feelings and sensations.

Next comes our active defence responses, flight and fight (mobilisation).

What happens when you've been working with a sharp implement and accidentally dropped it towards your bare feet? In a split-second, you move your foot out of the way. This is your flight system in action.

I once walked to the front door of a restaurant and saw three men beating another man on the ground with a weapon. Fifty people were watching and doing nothing. I yelled out to them, "STOP IT!" This was my fight system in action. Trust me, when the abusers started walking towards me, my whole body wanted to run (flight), but I overrode it to stay and face the consequences. (A combination of fight/flight/freeze).

You will have experienced these reactions through arguments and running away from challenging situations.

Fight-flight-freeze responses are not conscious decisions. They're automatic reactions that generate many physiological changes in the body. Each reaction begins in the amygdala, the part of your brain responsible for perceiving threats, real or imagined. It then sends a message to your hypothalamus, which stimulates the ANS.

How you will react is determined by the threat, your previous life experiences and the current state of your nervous system. The organising principle of life in your mind-body system determines your necessary survival protection response.

When your ANS is mobilised for survival, your brain sends the chemical communication for your body to immediately release the stress hormones, thus creating physiological changes.

If your body is always under threat, real or perceived, the continual changes impact your life. And when it's constantly mobilised, it's like driving with one foot on the accelerator and one on the brake simultaneously. You're burning through a lot of energy and yet not going anywhere.

Consider that constant mobilisation will impact your sleep, digestion, hormones, skin, vitality, energy, circulation, blood pressure, heart, and all of your relationships, as the energy is being used for protection.

Here are some of the ways this happens:

Physical	Emotional	Relational	Productivity
Chronic Fatigue	Depression	Toxic Relationships	Resistance
Obesity	Anxiety	Going blank in the middle of a conversation	Procrastination
Heart Disease	Overwhelm	Inability to set boundaries	Brain Fog
Stroke	Fear of Failure	Longing for intimacy but unable to attain it	Perfectionism
Insomnia	Fear of Success	Lack of empathy	Overachiever
Gut Challenges	Panic Attacks	No desire to connect or bond with others	Playing Small
Chronic Pain	Low self-esteem and self-worth (inaccurate)	Parenting Struggles	Not being able to achieve what you know is possible
Adrenal Fatigue	Hopelessness	Not being seen	Trouble asking for help
Addiction	Helplessness	Not being heard	No sense of purpose

What do you think people's biggest problems in life are?

Our biggest problem is misalignment with who and what we really are, which leads to disconnection. It starts with a dis-regulated nervous system. With the evolution to mammals, the ANS evolved to include a social engagement aspect. This brings the capacity for connection and co-regulation as an addition to the fight-flight-freeze responses of the ANS. We have this capacity to be with ourselves and others, which brings forth a desire and the freedom to connect. We need it like we need air and water.

Misalignment and disconnection are linked to the state of our nervous system.

As young children, we've all had intense, overwhelming experiences and feelings. Research now reveals the vital importance of having at least one significant relationship to teach the infant child how to co-regulate their nervous system as a precursor to being able to self-regulate. If that didn't happen, the child's capacity to do this would be diminished.

Your early experiences shape your nervous system, which means if it's not regulated, your nervous system will shape/create you.

So, what happens when your nervous system does create you? It means that you may be stuck in

- freeze (leading to depression)
- flight (leading to anxiety)
- fight (leading to toxic/violent/abusive relationships, or none at all)
- a combination of survival modes.

If you learn early in life to co-regulate, you can, no matter what, easily bring yourself back to equilibrium and your true values. This generates the capacity to focus the highest aspects of your mental, physical and emotional bodies towards building your dreams and goals, while living your life connected and on purpose.

The most distressing part about being locked in the three modes of survival is that you disconnect from who and what you really are, and who you fundamentally are is an extraordinary being of love connected on many dimensions. You're a potent creator who can manifest anything by focussing with the highest intention on the mental body, combined with the powerful fuel of the emotional body, and bringing it into form with the present-moment awareness of the physical body.

If you disconnect from who you really are, you're misaligned from the source of your energy and passion, and from the organising principle of your life. This means the quality of health, relationships and success you're able to generate is greatly reduced.

What's the worst thing that's ever happened to you, and how did you overcome it?

There's a photo of me in our backyard. It's my fifth birthday, and I'm blowing out the candles. Over my left shoulder, you can see the corner of a prison cell. The police station was attached to the house. My father, the local policeman, was often called out to disturbances, and he never knew how many people, with or without weapons, would be lying in wait to assault him. It wasn't until years after we left this town that my father didn't jump when the phone rang, and it took many decades before we realised he'd been suffering from PTSD.

My childhood environment was one of high stress, distress and tension. The people coming to the house or police station were experiencing challenging circumstances and were upset or aggressive. The body is always looking to create a sense of equilibrium. My normal was a world of distressed victims and perpetrators, so over time, my internal barometer increased to a new normal.

As a result, I did the only thing that felt natural to me, which was to get into a career within the criminal justice system.

My early childhood experiences shaped my nervous system, and then my nervous system shaped me. I spent seventeen years growing up within sight of the police station and prison cell, in addition to my twenty-five years working as the Registrar/Chamber Magistrate of the Court House, with every client presenting in a state of distress or tension. For forty years, I operated with a nervous system that spent most of its time in survival protection mode. From a lack of feeling safe, I created an overachiever/doer personality with hidden beliefs of "I am not safe" and "I am not enough".

Now, those survival protection mechanisms are vitally important, because otherwise, our species would have died out a long time ago. The problem starts when the mechanism is switched on constantly (not feeling safe), at times it doesn't have to be (when you really are safe), so a regulated nervous system becomes dis-regulated.

This is not to say that I didn't have social and connected moments or experience times of friendship, freedom and fun. What I'm saying is that many of those moments were built on a foundation of survival and pretence. My nervous system was already mobilised for protection without sufficient release, and then constant internal and external pressure was added daily through my work functions. The extreme amount of stress and tension I experienced, in addition to the internal pressure I placed on myself, resulted in a greater disconnection and misalignment from my Self.

More and more, I would see people having fun in a way I couldn't. I was looking at life through a Perspex cage (freeze response), wondering why I couldn't be part of normal life. It was a gradual process of disconnection through the original misalignment. My body started to show it was in distress with skin and digestive issues, as well as insomnia. I reached out to our Employees Assistance Program when I was struggling at work, and they would send me home to read a book. I was doing yoga and meditating, what I'd been told were all the right activities to deal with stress, but I was gradually getting even more exhausted mentally, physically and emotionally.

Finally, the dam burst.

I didn't understand the survival protection pattern of being an overachiever, so I believed the internal voice when it told me "I wasn't good enough". In order not to feel shame, I pushed my body long past its limit. I didn't listen to the signals it was sending. I suppressed my emotions, until my body screamed, "ENOUGH!" I hit rock bottom mentally, physically, emotionally and spiritually, and was forcibly retired on medical grounds. After being diagnosed with Complex PTSD, burn out, chronic fatigue, depression and anxiety, I had a one in five chance of ever working again.

My life had come to a grinding halt. It was a dark, hard place, and I remained there for a long time. Finding my way, and having the courage to say *yes* to things that seemed like a real risk at first, gave me a deep gratitude for the strength of my spirit.

After hearing the diagnosis and watching my life change dramatically, I said, "If I can never work again, I will become the healthiest person I possibly can as my contribution to the planet".

Unbeknownst to me, I'd accidentally engaged one of the higher faculties of the mind. I had no idea at the time the power of that intention and the life-giving adventure it would set me on. I needed to start at the beginning to learn the power of the mind and how to manage emotions, listen to the wisdom of the body and become aligned with my soul, my Self and Source. It wasn't until I healed at the level of the nervous system, that the foundations of vitality and vibrancy I'd only caught glimpses of, became rock solid.

How did you become interested in the nervous system?

Do you remember the story of *The Three Little Pigs*?

A strong breath would blow down the houses of straw and sticks, but nothing could destroy the house made of bricks.

Healing at the level of the nervous system builds the house of bricks.

I'd tried everything to heal by participating in many modalities all around the world. However, after all of my hard work, I would have a small reprieve before something would blow my house down again. Then one day, synchronicity had me living in Phoenix, Arizona, and someone gave me a book about how the body also needs to tell the story through nervous system regulation. That book, *The Revolutionary Trauma Release Process* by Dr David Berceli, was the final piece in the puzzle.

I understood why I kept reliving patterns of behaviour that were bringing dis-ease rather than vitality. It made me take a closer look at the survival protection responses and how they related to everyday life, mentally, physically and emotionally.

1. **Freeze (Immobilised)**
    We may not currently have to fight the elements to maintain our survival, however freeze responses today may look like the following:

    *   **Immobilisation or containment**
        Not saying what needs to be said (going completely blank) or finding it hard to express anything at all.

    *   **Feeling numb most of the time**
        Experiencing little desire or ability to be social.

- **Not having access to higher mental functions**
  Not being able to move forward in the direction of your dreams or goals. There's no access to passion or purpose. They're deadened, just like the capacity to feel happiness, joy or delight.

- **Remaining motionless**
  Having no energy to do or feel anything.

2. **Flight (Mobilised)**
Symptoms of flight include the following:

- Pretending a situation didn't happen.
- Avoiding confrontation (even leaving the room to avoid it).
- Cleaning the house instead of doing the assignment or project.
- Changing geographical locations, thinking it will change the situation.

3. **Fight (Mobilised)**
Fight can be activated in situations like a stressful day at work or being in congested traffic, and include the following:

- Having disproportionate flashes of anger or frustration to any given situation.
- Being defensive, even when you know your point of view has no merit.
- Being aggressive to those you love.

Consider anxiety as being locked in flight mode. It happens when you feel that a future-based activity could be dangerous or stressful, or you can't stop thinking about an event that happened in the past.

I'll give you an example. I went skydiving once, which put me in a combination of all the survival modes. While I was going through the motions of preparing for the jump, sitting in the open doorway of the plane, I saw the ground a long way below and had the sense of being completely out of sync. I was attempting to follow directions and get my body to go into the right positions, and yet it was like moving and thinking through molasses.

I may have had a smile plastered on my face, however internally, I was like a rabbit in the headlights, frozen in one spot. The smile was to ensure my fear was well hidden from others, including myself. I remember wondering what was happening. Why was my body not moving, when my mind was telling it to? Then the instructor pushed me out. No more time to think before I was flying through the air with an incredible present-moment flow state, a balance between the sympathetic and parasympathetic systems. 'Play' is another name for this state!

An hour after the jump, while in the car on the way to lunch, my thoughts went into a crazy anxiety overdrive as I thought of all the things that could have gone wrong. This was a dis-regulated nervous system in action. I was back on the ground, physically safe, but I didn't feel that way. My mind was attempting to think its way to safety, as the delayed effects of the terror came to the surface.

What happens in your day-to-day life can provide clear information as to what aspect of your nervous system (connection or protection) is running the show. Does it easily move from one state to the other when needed? You can recognise it through the use of your words, thoughts, actions, beliefs and attitudes. During my healing journey, this is what I experienced. What resonates with you?

Danger Level	State	Attitudes Beliefs and Behaviours	Thoughts of:	Feelings and Felt Senses
Life Threat	Freeze: The oldest and highest defence aspect of the nervous system. It comes from single-cell marine life, whose protection was to remain motionless and feign death.	On autopilot. Watching life pass you by through a screen. The world is like a movie, and I'm not in it. Like a rabbit in the headlights. Fear that can be well-hidden through the mask of smiling and pretending. Forgetful Spaced-out Losing track of time. You're untrustworthy, so I must depend on myself.	Hopelessness Shamefulness Humiliation Everyone else has their life together. I must be the only reject. Things don't seem real. Catastrophic thinking.	Numb Exhausted Depressed Trapped Unworthy Scattered

Danger Level	State	Attitudes Beliefs and Behaviours	Thoughts of:	Feelings and Felt Senses
Danger	Flight	Not able to remain still. Always doing things for others. Not being able to say no. Panicked The world is indifferent and unreliable. Being hyper-focussed on getting it right and saying the right thing. Being hypervigilant	Anxiety Worrisome thoughts Fearful thoughts 'What if' thoughts	Fast heart rate Shallow breathing Mobilised (tensed) and ready to move. High-pitched strained voice Excitable
Danger	Fight	Controlling Aggressive Overbearing Hurting others Hating others	I will hurt/fight/ attack you. How dare you! I hate you.	Tension Bracing Resistance Boiling emotions Annoyed Angry Frustrated

Danger Level	State	Attitudes Beliefs and Behaviours	Thoughts of:	Feelings and Felt Senses
Feeling safe	Freedom to be, connect and be social.	I can soothe myself. I can manage my emotions. The world is my oyster. Creative Collaborative Curious Compassionate Present Content	There's always a way. Loving and kind I am not my emotions.	Open Joyful Connected Embodied Safe Settled Grounded Regular heartbeat Deep lower-belly breathing Variation in vocal pitch and tone

I don't recommend a rock-bottom journey. What I do recommend is that you take note of which state of the nervous system you find yourself in most of the time, and if you're easily able to bring yourself back from protection to connection.

My diagnosis was simultaneously the worst and best thing that ever happened to me. It gave me the path home to being aligned and connected to myself, so I could shine a light for others.

What is your big WHY?

I've always been passionate about the magic of communication. There's this moment when you get the power of language, when you know you can create anything and influence anyone to collaborate and connect with you.

Quantum physicists indicate that everything is energy. It's always transmuting and changing. A thought is energy. You can't have anything without it. If you're locked into a specific survival aspect of your nervous system, you will be fixed in your ways of being, thinking and feeling in ways that don't support communication and connection.

This happens on a micro scale with individuals, and on a macro scale with corporations, organisations, countries and governments. The health of your nervous system, and your capacity to connect and communicate on an individual level, also has an impact on a global level.

ANS	Communications Behaviours	Self	Loved Ones	Countries	Corporations
Freeze	Withholding love Not saying what needs to be said.	Not being able to say no or set boundaries.	Withholding love Resentment	Sanctions	Squeeze out or freeze out
Flight	Withdrawing from connection Isolation	Gotta get out of here.	Making excuses Leave when conversations get tough.	Refugees and asylum seekers	Liquidation Bankruptcy
Fight	Arguments and fighting	Self-hatred conversations Telling yourself you're not good enough	Arguments and fighting	Wars	Hostile takeovers
Safe	Connecting with love	Self-love and compassion	Connecting with love, kindness and compassion	Peace Co-operation Collaboration	Win/win/win for everyone.

There are so many people in the world struggling with some challenge or another, whether it's on a personal, community or global level. I desire to help people understand that everything that happens to an individual, also impact friends, families, communities and the world at large. Healing at the level of an individual's nervous system has the power to dramatically change their life and the world, one body at a time.

Every aspect of your being communicates. All communication within yourself, with yourself and with others, internally or externally, has an impact on your health and success, your capacity to love and be loved, your community, and ultimately, your world.

It's my mission and passion to support people in becoming aligned, connected and fluent in the languages of their being, so they can live their true life. Every single person has wisdom to share when they listen from the most connected part of themselves. From this place, there's only win/win/win...for self, for others and for the world.

My legacy, my big Why, is sharing this work with the world, so we can all take personal responsibility for the state of our own nervous system and our planet, and live an extraordinary life on our own terms.

Why was discovering the importance of the nervous system such a powerful moment in your own healing journey?

I had done a lot of healing work on the physical, mental, emotional and spiritual aspects of myself, yet I would still have these overreactions and startled responses, and I continued to experience symptoms of insomnia, poor digestion, fatigue, procrastination and lack of desire for social interaction.

I had this intuitive thought that told me, *There's fear in my body.* The power of the intention I'd set years earlier went into motion.

Synchronicity kicked in, as it had done many times before. After reading Dr Berceli's book, I could see my life through his journey. Not the content, but the context of it. So I was delighted to find out Dr Berceli was teaching in my city the following weekend. Becoming a certified practitioner of the Trauma Release Process (TRE), was the beginning of my deep-dive into the nervous system and the foundation of my regained health, energy, relationships and success on my terms.

Each aspect of our brain-body being needs to release the story mentally, emotionally and physically. My body had not yet released the adrenalised survival responses, which are stored as muscular tension or trauma patterns. The moments of overwhelm, intensity, fear and terror, if not processed by the nervous system in the moment, remain in the body, until they can be processed or resolved at some later date.

Our lives are so busy, we don't make the time to resolve the past, until a crisis hits. Those tension and trauma patterns bring pain and discomfort, in addition to precursor symptoms to life threatening diseases. These patterns limit our success, beliefs, thoughts, actions and capacity to give and receive love. They also restrict our ability to regulate emotional outbursts and our behaviours towards connection or protection.

It doesn't matter if the trauma or tension is from single events or intense stress over long periods of time. Research now tells us that a personality rearranges itself to fit inside the changed physiology of a body that holds trauma or tension. In other words, limitations appear in every aspect of your being and world. If not processed immediately, what could have been a short-term solution for a short-term problem, becomes a long-term problem, as it has rewired neural pathways in your brain.

Have you ever wondered why these challenging situations or patterns in your life continue to reoccur in relationships, workplace bullying situations and business failures? The state of your nervous system determines the story you're telling yourself about living within those aspects of life that are important to you.

When your autonomic nervous system mobilises a fight/flight or immobilisation-freeze response, your brain releases a chemical communication into the muscles. If those communications aren't completely utilised in the survival response, they're stored in the body. Your mind/body system, aligned with the organising principle of life, will continue to create similar circumstances for you to survive and thrive from that event. This happens, so you can discharge the adrenalised energy and process that previous situation.

Once the discharge happens, the limitations in your mind (fixed mindset), your body (lack of presence and connection), emotions (overwhelm) and behaviours, are also released.

The end result is that your alignment, intention, presence and fuel become available for your passions, purpose and dreams.

As previously mentioned, your autonomic nervous system affects your organs and glands, as well as the systems in your body. If you're having symptoms, consider that they've been impacted by a nervous system response that hasn't been brought back to balance, and is therefore impacting the energy available for your healing or your life. Until you deal with it at the level of the nervous system, you won't make a lasting impact on your energy. This in turn impacts your capacity for great relationships and lasting success, as well as your health, vitality and wellbeing, all things I know are important to you.

Have you ever seen a jellyfish in water? It expands and contracts as it moves through life. It's a fully alive, pulsating organism in its natural environment. You're the same. And just like the jellyfish, you need both expansion and contraction to navigate your environment. The problem arises when you're stuck in contraction mode, unable to move easily and rhythmically between the two. Locked into protection or contraction, surviving not thriving, is the only option available.

As a species, we've forgotten and suppressed our body's innate intelligence and capacity to regulate itself after a survival response. However, it is possible to regain that knowledge.

How are you currently making a difference in other people's lives?

I help people become aligned with who and what they really are, heal their nervous system for a greater capacity to receive, release the past and create the future that is waiting for them.

Do you have a special system you use to help people?

I've created the 7 Steps to Becoming Aligned system to help people come back to the truth and magnificence of who they really are by releasing the past, so it no longer defines the present or the future.

Step One: Awareness for Clarity

You build awareness to clarify where you are and where you wish to go. Everything you do in life is playing the gap between where you are and your desires.

"Awareness is all about restoring your freedom to choose what you want, instead of what your past imposes on you."
~ Deepak Chopra

Step Two: Learn Your Languages

To become fluent in the languages of your being, you need to become aware of them. Words, thoughts, beliefs, attitudes, emotions, felt perceptions and sensations, are all communications.

Listening and mapping these communications will tell you in which state of your nervous system you spend most of your time and how to shift into its correct hierarchy, with social engagement at the top.

Step Three: Ignite Your Vision

The quickest path to burnout and overwhelm is attempting to live the life of someone else. It impairs your work performance and severely impacts your vitality and wellbeing.

It's time to be engaged and energised by living your true life and reconnecting with the deepest desires and visions of your spirit. Reignite your intuition and imagination, and utilise your higher mental faculties to hold your intention front and centre.

Step Four: Generate Your Genius, Grace and Gifts

Genius is a potential that lives within you and every other human being. The ability to master the mind (intention), the body (presence) and the emotions (fuel), will supply you with everything you need to develop the habits of generating your own genius, grace and gifts. The Universal source called intention (genius), is connected to everything and everyone, and is available for unique expression through you.

> "Everyone is born a genius, but the process of
> living de-geniuses them."
> ~ Buckminster Fuller

Step Five: Navigate Your Plan

If you can conceive it, you can achieve it. A goal/dream or vision needs a plan. Your capacity to map your nervous system will help you activate your internal GPS, your intuition and your capacity to know what you need and take action, as the vision of your life guides you.

Step Six: Expand and Embody Your Capacity to Receive

Life is about embodying presence. The more present you can become, the more you'll be able to respond in the moment, and the greater your capacity to receive all of the blessings that are available for you.

Step Seven: Develop Your Desires

The physical body has this powerful relationship with desire that, when used correctly, creates an amazing magnetism that just brings your people, places, circumstances, situations and things into your path for your next step. Then it can be used to empower synchronicity.

How else are you currently making a difference in other people's lives?

I work specifically to support people in healing their nervous system and releasing trauma and tension patterns stored in the body after natural disasters or intense workplace crises. Currently, I'm working with emergency services personnel, police and firefighters, so they can discharge the adrenalised energy and reconnect with themselves and loved ones.

I'm also supporting people who were affected by the 2019-2020 Australian Summer bushfires to regain their balance and equilibrium as they rebuild their communities.

Do you have any final words to share?

All of our words, thoughts, stories, actions and behaviours are governed by the state of our nervous system and our capacity to move between connection and protection when necessary. Being stuck in protection mode, your energy is focussed on survival, with no capacity to thrive. It's possible to release the past and utilise the powerful energy that illuminates all of who you are, for a life that is truly yours. You can live aligned and generate authentic happiness, meaning, fulfilment, success, love and connection on your terms. Elevating your energy!

My greatest desire is for everyone to know it's possible to have the health, energy, vitality, deep connection and success they choose, when they attain a well-regulated nervous system.

To discover more about how Karen can help you *Elevate Your Energy*, simply visit www.elevatebooks.com/energy

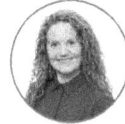

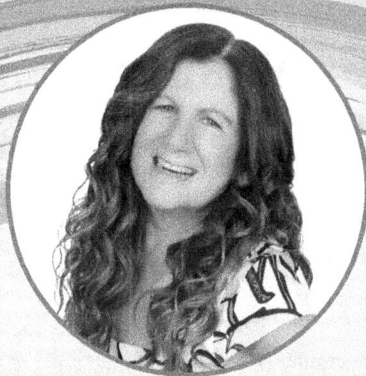

Leonie Shanahan

Your Health is Your Wealth

Leonie is a professional speaker, workshop facilitator, health coach and columnist for *Organic Gardener* magazine. She's also the founder of the Edible School Gardens program and is the author of *Lyme Disease Sucks: the trauma, the truth & the triumph.*

Her 7 Pillars of Health program helps people detox in all areas of their life, challenge their perceptions and live their purpose.

Leonie changes lives by helping people delete negative emotional and physical habits, so they become empowered, vibrantly healthy, energetic and joyful. Her passion, energy and absolute love of life is a result of surviving her Lyme journey and teaching others how to fully love their life and thrive.

Leonie Shanahan

Your Health is Your Wealth

What fears did you have to overcome at the start of your journey?

The day I got my Lyme results back from the U.S.A., my whole world crashed. I was terrified. My doctor was talking to me about treatment, but I couldn't hear a word she was saying. I was numb and so scared. I didn't know how, or even if, I would get through this illness. As a single mum, I was at a loss as to how I was going to be able to care for my daughter. How was I going to cook, and get her to school, and just function with the antibiotic treatment that would make me so sick? Although I'd been researching about Lyme leading up to the results, I'd still hoped it would be a negative, so I was in shock when I received the diagnosis.

After remaining in the foetal position in bed for a couple of days, I reminded myself that I was good with projects. I thrive on them. I just had to find a natural way to get well, so I could then help others get well too. I needed to contact people in other countries that treated Lyme and ask how they did it, buy up any books on the subject and search the internet for health professions in the world who had positive solutions.

With my new goal and new purpose, I took my first vital steps out of bed to work on the most difficult, expensive and challenging project I'd ever undertaken, but also the most important, since my life depended on it. There's so much controversy surrounding the disease with it not even being recognised in Australia. It's criminal, as there are hundreds of thousands of people in Australia alone trying to navigate the speed bumps of regaining their health. The support from the medical system is cruelly inconsequential. Most doctors don't even know how to recognise or treat it, so they often tell their sick patients that it's in their heads. But even if you do find a doctor who treats Lyme, your symptoms have to be called 'Lyme-like'.

Lyme disease is real, and my multi-year journey has taken me through a mirage of treatments. In desperation, like most Lyme patients, I've risked trying anything to look for relief from my various debilitating symptoms. Though I was eventually successful, it was a slow journey that often felt like one step forward, ten steps back.

What is Lyme disease?

Lyme disease is an infectious illness caused by the bacterium known as Borrelia, which creates a condition more correctly known as Borreliosis.

The bacteria, a spirochete (a flexible spirally-twisted bacterium), is transmitted when an individual is bitten by a vector, usually a tick, but it can also be mosquitoes, sandflies and cat fleas. Lyme disease can impact many bodily systems and organs, and is often called 'the great imitator', as it takes on the properties of other illnesses, such as MS, chronic fatigue, lupus and Alzheimer's.

People with Lyme disease are frequently diagnosed with other co-infections caused by vector-borne bacteria and parasites, such as Babesia, Bartonella, Rickettsia, Mycoplasma and Ehrlichia.

The disease is multi-layered and complicated. There are over 144 different symptoms, and they change as the disease moves around your body. Lyme and its co-infections don't have a set pathway, which makes it more difficult to treat patients, as there isn't a one-treatment-fits-all approach.

There are ways to tell if you have early- or late-stage Lyme disease.

▶ Early stages of Lyme disease
When you first get bitten, the early signs are usually flu-like symptoms with fevers, fatigue, swollen glands, sore throat, nausea and vomiting, headaches, stiff neck, muscle aches, joint pain, light sensitivity and neurological symptoms. Seek treatment immediately to stop the disease from getting inside your cells.

▶ Late-stage Lyme disease
Late-stage Lyme disease can last for years, often manifesting as a multi-systemic illness which may include gastro-intestinal, neurological and balance problems, as well as chronic fatigue and random muscle and joint pain. There are so many symptoms. Late-stage Lyme disease can be mild, moderate or severe, and if left untreated can cause acute disability or become fatal.

How did you recover?

First, I had to want to recover, which isn't a choice everyone makes. I had a reason to live and set about getting to that end goal, but I had no roadmap to get there. In fact, being in Australia, you're basically on your own most of the time trying to get through the quicksand of bureaucracy. I had to seek out my own core support team of friends to help guide me, as my brain fog and ability to see beyond today was seriously challenged. My team was there to remind me of my purpose and be my cheer squad to keep me going. I had to prioritise self-love and receiving help from others.

I also had a team of health professionals that understood disease and were willing to research to find out more. It took a long time to find them, as many refuse to even admit Lyme disease exists in Australia. My main team consists of doctors, a kinesiologist, a Bioresonance practitioner, a Chinese medicine/acupuncture practitioner, a lymphatic massage therapist, a colonic therapist, a cranial-sacral therapist and a reiki practitioner. Supplements and exercise add an essential boost.

What are your 7 Pillars of Health?

These are the 7 pillars of health that I brought into my life to heal, each entwining with the others. They rebuild the mind, body and spirit, so you can become an even better version of yourself. Your true you will emerge, as all the layers of the onion will have shredded. I teach them through workshops and zoom.

▸ **Pillar 1: Drop the Stress**
Find the causes of your stress, and learn coping strategies to replace it with positive action/thought/story. One example is to use your breath to calm you. Breathe in slowly for five seconds, hold for six, release very slowly for seven. Get outside, and if possible, spend time in nature.

▸ **Pillar 2: Detox All Areas of Your Life**
Detox toxic relationships with your

- partner
- friends
- work
- children
- yourself.

Detox your body with

- a body brush
- saunas
- coffee enemas
- colonics
- foot baths
- Epsom salt/bicarbonate of soda baths.

Detox your mind by clearing out all of the clutter/negative chat that doesn't serve you. Techniques include

- decluttering your home
- clearing out old memories.

▶ **Pillar 3: Sleep Hygiene**
If you don't get a good night's sleep, your body can't heal, your brain can't detox and you'll be unable to function. Make sure you're aware of your sleep hygiene practices, your circadian rhythms, and have definite pre-bed rituals, so your body understands it's time for rest.

▶ **Pillar 4: Grow and Eat Organic Food**
Your health is your wealth, and it starts with growing your own organic food in your backyard in soils that are *alive*. Organic food that brings health, strength, vitality and healing. Food that brings you towards health and never towards dis-ease.

▶ **Pillar 5: Chemical-Free Living**
Clean out your pantry, bathroom, bedroom, lounge room, office and car of anything that emits harmful chemicals.

▶ **Pillar 6: Vagus Activation**
The vagus is communicating from the brain to the gut, and back again, including all of your organs in that area. It's an incredibly important nerve that needs to be activated during the day. Do your research to learn fun ways to activate it.

▶ **Pillar 7: Living Your Purpose**
This has to do with visualisation, intentions, setting goals, diary writing, accountability and education.

Elevate Your Energy

What do you think are the biggest obstacles you've had to deal with due to having Lyme disease?

For me, it's not only the mega-bundle of challenges, but also all of the co-infections and possible side effects.

There's also the huge amount of grief associated with the loss of my Edible School Garden business that I absolutely loved, and the loss of identity and income that went along with it.

I had to say goodbye to my much loved home and organic property, as well as to a lot of friends. People stop wanting to be around you when you're less able to physically do what you used to. Because you don't look sick, they expect you to function as normal and may be intolerant when you can't keep up, so they stop asking you to go places.

As a mother, I'd always handled everything, so when I suddenly couldn't, it was hard to ask for help.

What's the biggest mistake people make when they're exhausted and suffering with chronic Lyme?

People want to go in for the kill and wipe out the active Lyme, which is what I did as well, but there are multiple layers before your body and mind are ready to eradicate it.

First, you need to clear up all of the emotional baggage of life, including stress, trauma, depression and anxiety, anywhere from childhood to the present. You also need a Lyme-literate practitioner who will guide you through the mountain of supplements and tonics you will need.

Find your new tribe. They're the ones who will listen, love you, wipe your tears, hold you together when you need it, and if you're really lucky, provide healthy, organic meals, since your new diet will be no grains, dairy, alcohol, sugar or junk food.

What are your tips for getting through this difficult time?

With depression, as with Lyme, you suffer terribly for multiple reasons. I set ground rules for myself after the first time I wanted to end my life. If I'm still depressed after three days, I go and seek professional help as soon as possible, as I've learned that after this time, I no longer have any capacity to help myself, and I'm heading downstream quickly.

When you're in a state of anger and hopelessness, it's good to contact someone supportive. They should preferably be local, so they can monitor you throughout the day. Make sure it's someone you feel safe with who understands, so you can feel free to vent your anger.

It's important to make yourself get out of bed. Try putting on brightly coloured clothes and being around other people. Often the very act of removing yourself from your home and placing yourself in completely different surroundings can lift you enough to start functioning again in a more positive way. Even if it only elevates your mood slightly, it's something you can build upon.

Spending time in nature is so important. Mother Nature is there to nurture and hold you. Lying on a blanket and looking at the clouds is helpful. Let your mind focus on something besides your situation.

If no one is home, get a pool noodle or other soft stick-like object, and hit a pillow as hard as you can while screaming. Get all of your frustration and anger *out* of your body. Keep hitting that pillow until it's released. You have got to get the anger out.

Try driving in your car and screaming your lungs out on a deserted road. Another favourite I've done for years when I get annoyed, and there are people around, is that I go into the toilet, screw up my face and tense my whole body, including my fists, as long and hard as I can, and then end it with a silent lion's roar. It releases all of the tension out of your body. It's soooo good.

Go for a walk or do some gardening. Get your hands in the soil. Play with an animal.

Watch or listen to a comedy.

Make sure you have a caring practitioner who's checking all of your blood work for chemical imbalances. Keep searching for ones who understand how difficult your current health crisis is. Giving out antidepressants like they're candy, isn't the answer. We need loving support, understanding, direction and supplements.

There is a huge range of treatments available to support your body that are listed in my book *Lyme Disease Sucks: the trauma, the truth & the triumph.*

What I suggest for Lyme people will also be relevant to anyone with a chronic illness or who wants to ensure they stay healthy with a strong immunity.

What activities do you participate in that you never would have dreamed about doing as the previous you?

It seems when you have a health crisis, suddenly every orifice is a new inlet for deeper healing!!

I don't even drink coffee, I've always hated the smell. I could never imagine that I would be inserting it into my body with coffee enemas and colonics.

I also use a Neti pot to clear my nasal cavity.

I did a three-month car holiday, driving from Queensland through NSW and Victoria. It felt so expansive and brave for me, as I was still quite unwell. I loved my time alone, constantly stopping to enjoy whatever filled my love cup – like massive trees, pelicans on the lake, swans with signets, a spring farm, baby animals, botanical gardens, festivals and … nothingness. I absorbed nature, completely in awe of her undying beauty.

What can someone do for a loved one who has a chronic illness?

- Cook while being mindful of their diet restrictions.
- Clean for them.
- Hug them.
- Make them feel nurtured.
- Fluff up their pillow.
- Tuck a blanket around, so they feel secure.
- Let them know it's okay for them to go back to bed as soon as they feel tired.
- Watch a movie/favourite show with them.
- Ask what you can do to show them you love them.
- Write notes about why you love them.
- Drive them somewhere in nature, even if you both just sit in the car and gaze out the window.
- Celebrate every milestone, no matter how small.
- Be their best cheerleader.
- Remind them of their future self.
- Allow them to express their emotions. Listen with an open heart, without comment or judgment.
- Be patient and have compassion. They're suffering with multiple symptoms, both physical and emotional.
- Remember that they need you.

How do you start your day?

Mornings are precious for my mind and body. I naturally wake at dawn and bathe in the joy of birdsong. Before I get out of bed, I ask my angels if there are any messages for me that may have come from my dreams. Then I do the following:

- Give multiple gratitudes. For example, I give thanks for the sun shining, a good night's sleep, my strong legs, and water to have a shower.
- Visualise my day playing out the way I want it, in a mini movie.
- Get out of bed.
- Do a tongue scraping.
- Do oil pulling, which draws toxins out of the mouth and improves the health of my gums and teeth. It feels so good.
- Use a Neti pot nasal rinse four or five times a week. It may seem strange at first, pouring liquid though your nostrils like some party trick, but stay with it, as it totally clears your sinuses!
- Gaggle some water.
- Throw cold water onto my face.
- Go outside to ground myself (barefoot), and let the sunshine onto my face.
- Do a meditation where I imagine I'm holding a bright orange ball cradled in my outstretched hand, and inside of it is all my dreams, my future, and what I want to achieve in life. Then I crouch down and give the ball to the earth for her to make my dreams come true.
- Do some warm-up stretches, a little yoga and then bounce on a lymphasizer trampoline.
- Pick my greens from the garden for the day's meals.
- Have breakfast, which consists of celery juice, a green smoothie and grain-free bread, along with a whole bunch of supplements.
- Check emails and messages.
- Get out into the sun for at least twenty minutes to build up Vitamin D.

What is your night-time routine?

I watch some comedy, because you can't have too many laughs in your life. I also turn off all computer/phone devices at least an hour before bed. If I've had a bad day and am not a happy camper, I write in my 'release' book. It's a journal where I chronicle all of the issues that are making me upset, worried or angry, and ask the angels to deal with them while I sleep. This journal does not live in my bedroom – my bedroom is for peace, love and sleep, with no devices or TV. I only keep my gratitude diary by my bed. Then I read a novel until I feel sleepy.

I sleep on a biomat, which is a healing pad of amethyst crystals, far-infrared rays and negative ions that repair your tissues and support your immune system. It also decreases pain and detoxes me.

Where does your passion for growing food come from?

When my first daughter was born, I made a promise to her that my next job would make a difference in the world. At the time, I was working in optical and hated it. I thought about my values and passions. I'd spent a lot of time travelling overseas before I became a mum, and people in third-world countries had a special place in my heart, because of their generosity and happy, kind and joyful spirit.

I decided to study horticulture. I liked growing food, so I figured I could become qualified and then work in Cambodia where they'd lost a generation of farmers and needed a boost to their agriculture. It took six years to qualify, as I only did a couple of subjects at a time as I had to be there for my growing family.

I continued to further my education in permaculture and organics. As my children started school, I noticed the junk other children had in their lunchboxes with lots of colour but nothing real. It was all in packages with no nutritional value for their growing brain, body, and mind.

That's when I decided to start the Edible School Gardens program. It ran for a minimum of one year in each primary school, where the students learned all about permaculture design and then came up with a garden design for their school. The community came together with the students, and we brought our design alive in a day. Over the next year, the students learnt by practising everything about growing food, from the what, where and how of seeds and plants, to creating 'living soil'. Our favourite day was the harvest celebration, where chefs or parents, along with the students, cooked meals from what the garden had produced.

We decorated the tables with flowers, tablecloths and cutlery. There were no disposables. It was all either donated or purchased from op shops and we ate off real plates or large mulberry or arrowroot leaves.

Classes would organise a wide variety of entertainment, like creating harvest songs or dances, playing with baby farm animals and a pumpkin-rolling competition. We'd also have our version of *MasterChef*, with people judging recipes. I could write a book about the fun we had during those days. The students were so proud of their garden. We grew the best-looking food, and they loved cooking and eating it.

Lots of parents went on to create their own vegetable patches under the guidance of their child. My four goals were to embed the skill of organic gardening, get children eating fresh food, protect our environment, and create community. It was enormously rewarding work. The program was successful and attracted lots of support from companies and media. I was acknowledged with many awards.

A film crew decided they wanted to make a DVD of my program, so they followed me around for eighteen months at about five different schools, recording my teaching and the students' involvement and comments. If you're interested in seeing the finished results, visit https://edibleschoolgardens.com.au.

I also wrote a book during this time, entitled *Eat Your Garden: Organic Gardening for Home and School*, that I'm quite proud of. It's filled with so much information. The idea was to produce a full-colour book with easy, clear instructions about all of the processes in the world of gardening – from compost, worm towers/baths and lolly plants, to a guide for using plants as medicine and starting community projects.

My latest book *is Lyme Disease Sucks: the trauma, the truth & the triumph.*

When I got Lyme disease, I had to walk away from my edible school gardens business. I literally couldn't put one foot in front of the other or remember any of my wonderful gardening processes, as most of my memory seemed to have been wiped out.

The book highlights my long and slow recovery, and the importance of having a clear goal of where you want to be at the end of your journey. I talk about the massive ebbs and flows of my emotional and physical health, all of the treatments I tried and the uphill battle of getting people to understand this baffling disease. In the end, not only did I achieve my goal, but as a person, as a woman, I've never felt so strong within myself regarding who I am, what I want in life and why I'm here.

Is there a connection between organic food and your general health?

Food knows how to heal our body, but we've forgotten, or been diverted away from, this ancient knowledge by corporate greed, financial gain and power. They've created a sickness industry, once again providing a huge monetary gain to shareholders at our expense. How have we allowed them to bastardise our (real) food?

The state of our health, especially for children today, is appalling. There are supermarkets full of food without nutrients. We need to remove junk food and sugary drinks that are readily available everywhere, even in schools. So much of non-organic agriculture is laced in glysophate (a cancer-causing poison), none of which is adding to our health and wellbeing.

Disease is a commodity, and our children are the unauthorised stakeholders of this club that causes autism, ADHD, diabetes, chronic illness, obesity, and later in life, infertility, just to name a few. Children are so vulnerable to all of these toxins being thrown at and into their bodies. It's a crime against humanity. With all the information we have available, we should have the healthiest generation of children, but instead they will die at a younger age than their parents.

We can take back control over our health by growing our own organic, nutrient-dense, nutrient-rich food. We need to create soil that's alive with microbes and minerals that will feed our plants the goodness they require to be strong, healthy and resilient. Then when we eat these life-giving plants, they will convert their nutritional bounty and strength *to* us. Most natural food has a specific part of our body it supports and minerals to distribute, and often tries to provide us with clues as to which part they sustain. For example, walnuts look like a brain, and yes, they support it. A tomato with its four chambers is good for the heart. Carrots are good for the eyes, and avocado strengthens the uterus. Food is information and direction for our bodies.

Every day we need to have a vast variety of food – not the junk in a packet that will take nutrients away from you – but real, fresh food. Growing your own is easy. You can grow a huge selection of herbs and greens, and each morning when harvesting your food for the day pick a bit of everything without effort. Within a week, it's easy to enjoy over a hundred different types of health-giving foods. Each meal should consist of a rainbow of colourful, fresh items on your plate, as colour is just as important as variety. Every mouthful you ingest shapes your consciousness. Food is powerful.

When you grow your own, your gratitude to the process is so much deeper. You plant a seed, and miraculously, a plant emerges for you and your family to enjoy. Before each meal, I say my version of a prayer where I give thanks for the healthy food I'm going to eat that will make my body stronger and healthier. When I harvest, as I pick each item, I talk to the plants, expressing gratitude for growing such healthy, abundant sustenance for me.

If you were speaking to your younger self, what advice would you give?

I wish that when I was younger, someone had told me I could achieve any goal I was passionate about. I just had to spend time digging deep into my heart and discovering what my future self wanted to do to make this world a better place.

Here's the advice I'd give my younger self:

- Education is the most valued asset you can have. Always read, listen, watch and be objective. Question everything for its truth.
- Seek out mentors. Have role models. Set high goals.
- Follow what you believe in.
- Don't allow males to stop you from doing what's important to you.
- Find your tribe. Don't waste time with people who bring you down.
- Have growth-oriented friends/workplaces/partners.
- Be a voice for the voiceless, such as the environment, refugees, indigenous people and those living in third-world countries.
- Learn the wisdom of your elders. Listen to your wise grandparents, uncles, aunties and neighbours.
- Don't party so hard!
- What other people think of you is none of your business.

What are some of your future goals?

I want to get a van and travel around, seeing more of Australia.

While travelling, I would like to stop at rural and remote towns and give workshops on health and gardening. I also want to bring awareness about Lyme disease and the importance of staying healthy.

I'd like to have a showcase/demo organic, sustainable and healthy property/retreat space, with buildings made of hempcrete in a picturesque natural setting.

I would love to have a big party to celebrate a birthday, because I haven't celebrated it for seven years, as I've slept through them all with fatigue. I think January 2022 is my celebration year.

I want to inspire other Lyme people to get well and start living life again, and let them know it will look different from before, but that it's okay.

I dream of being a professional speaker, spreading the word about healthy eating and living, and how it can heal the body, mind and spirit.

I long to speak on Brendan Burchard's stage and be interviewed by Marie Forleo.

Why is health so important?

All humans have toxins in them. Unfortunately, our world is polluted with chemicals. The lungs of our earth, our forests, are being destroyed without any respect for their life-giving value.

Babies are born with over 287 chemicals found in umbilical cord blood. Each day, women on average absorb over 168 chemicals, mostly through personal care products.

People have more stuff than ever, but they're not happier. They're lonely, isolated and depressed, with no passion, purpose, joy or energy, and little fulfilment.

Our bodies are sick, tired, infertile and sleep-deprived, and our healthy biology is collapsing. We eat food laced with chemicals and use products dowsed in them. All of it promotes disease and takes away our full potential to live, robbing our energy and life force.

Yet we don't question the whys and just expect it to be fixed. There's a general 'pill for an ill' mentality, with nobody going upstream to understand the reality of why we're abusing our bodies with the food we eat, the products we use, the toxic chemicals in our house and car or the pollution in the air from the factories.

We don't understand the negative effects of EMF and 5G, our thoughts and words and the drugs we take. We need to respect our body for the incredible vessel it is. It's so forgiving and ready to accept radical changes to rebuild itself back to health and functionality, which also means living life with so much more meaning and fulfilment. Nourishment is vital for our health. We need to reconnect with our body, mind and spirit. Life is too short to suffer.

We've forgotten what it feels like to wake up in the morning and feel brilliant. We've all settled for all right, when we should be excited about the day, taking great joy in listening to the birds singing, which causes us to sing, because life is good. We toss and turn when we should be having a good night's sleep, waking up feeling recharged and energised, our minds clear and focussed. Our potential is limitless.

Feed your body good food, supplements and exercise, and surround yourself with people of a high vibration, positive energy and love. Everything is possible. Every decision you make is taking you towards health and wellness. Life is good.

When you're healthy, doing what you love and being around your true tribe, you function at a high level, enveloped in your true purpose. And it's not hard, because you attract it, fully embracing life with laughter, joy, love, clarity, respect, compassion, generosity and adventure. You're opening the doors of opportunity way beyond your goals.

Do you have any final words of wisdom?

I love this quote from the book *The Choice* by Edith Eger:

> "I sat and studied the faces of every passing stranger. What I saw deeply moved me. I saw boredom, fury, tension, worry, confusion, discouragement, disappointment, sadness, and most troubling of all, emptiness. It made me very sad to see so little joy and laughter. Even the dullest moments of our lives are opportunities to experience hope, buoyancy, happiness. Mundane life is life, too. As is painful life, and stressful life. Why do we so often struggle to feel alive or distance ourselves from feeling life fully? Why is it such a challenge to bring life to life?"
> *~ Edith Eger*

Write your own prescription for *fun* and *living* activities you've wanted to do, and make sure you achieve one each week. You're number one, so love yourself first. Find your joy, happiness, love, kindness, energy and compassion. Have control over your food supply by growing some. Get out into sun. Spend time in nature. Breathe. Relax. Sing. Hum. Love life.

Your body is designed to heal. Find your true purpose, and dig deep into your untouched strengths and resilience, so you can rebuild yourself to be healthy and strong again. Be vulnerable to allowing expansion, and release what no longer serves you. Every day is an opportunity to hit the reset button. LIVE the life that you deserve, not the one others are paving for you. When you find and truly love yourself, you will shine.

If you do this, you'll soon discover that every minute of your life is precious, and you won't waste a minute of it!

Remember, your health is your wealth.

To discover more about how Leonie can help you *Elevate Your Energy*, simply visit www.elevatebooks.com/energy

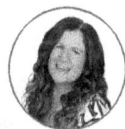

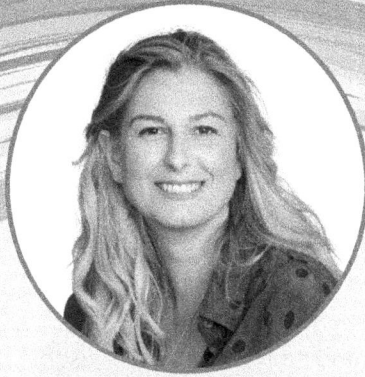

Marina Rei

A Whole-Hearted Life

Marina Rei is a transformational and leadership coach, meditation teacher, retreat host, speaker and entrepreneur. She also holds postgraduate degrees in education, counselling and international relations.

After twenty years of international work, study and research, Marina merged the wisdom of the East and West to create her Inner Healer and Inner Leader activation program that helps people fully step into their power, presence and purpose.

Marina is a true master at following her intuition and travels frequently. Her Master Within meditation course teaches deep meditation and transforms people's lives, personally and professionally.

Marina's private coaching empowers healers, teachers, entrepreneurs, leaders, seekers and impact-makers to realise their full potential, so they can create thriving relationships and businesses and live a meaningful life.

Marina Rei

A Whole-Hearted Life

How can people find their WHY?

The first and most important question you can ask yourself is...*Who am I?* Followed by the second most important question...*What is my why?*

You can meet thousands, even millions, of people, and no two answers will be the same. There are no identical fingerprints or blueprints for our lives. That is the beauty of our existence and self-discovery. We're unique with individual forms of expression, yet we're all created from the same divine energy.

2020 was a year when our personal and collective life structures were challenged. At times of global crisis, when there's so much uncertainty in and around us, we need to ask ourselves important questions about our identity, leadership and values. It's a time of reset and perhaps redefining our values, systems and structures.

During crisis, our primary emotion appears in the form of fear and separation, from ourselves and others. When we're in this state of fear or trauma, we're much more likely to lose our centre, which is our connection to ourselves. We can feel separate from the world we live in, yet we're also an active participant in it, whether we're aware of it or not.

But while there's fear, separation and isolation, at the same time, there's also an opportunity to go deeper within ourselves to connect with our truth, our power and our purpose, and also unify our fields of energy with love.

When Covid started, we could see and hear everywhere, "We're in this together!" And the truth is, we are! If we take as our truth that we all live on the same planet, coexisting and co-creating together, wouldn't it be invaluable if we took responsibility for our life force and our contribution to the world?

As cliché as it may sound, we all seek to feel loved, and self-love is a path to loving others, regardless of our differences. I'm inviting you to look at your life and see where you'd like more love, forgiveness and acceptance. Ask yourself, *Am I kind and loving towards myself? Who am I, and who am I becoming? Is this my truth?*

If you're willing to go on a journey of self-discovery to know your truth, your challenges have the potential to expand your soul. Moreover, these experiences are a doorway to finding your purpose and will reveal the area of impact where you can make a difference in other people's lives.

From my work and research, I can say that the most fulfilling, magnetic and energised people are those who know their Why and their purpose. They live life in alignment with their values and contribute to the wellbeing of others.

When people find their spiritual home and believe there's something greater than themselves, they begin to understand that we're all connected to our innate power and life force, and they transcend what they perceive as their failures.

"Your life is not a failure. You are a unique masterpiece in creation!"

What are you passionate about?

I've realised that it's more important than ever to teach and assist people how to connect with their truth, their energy, their power and their heart centre. I felt I had to take responsibility for my part and use my skills and wisdom to contribute and make a difference.

At times, it hasn't been easy to be seen for who I am and stand in my power and light. I felt I needed to step out of my comfort zone and leave my 'small self' behind. I had to put myself out there more and overcome my fears, so I could serve even more. Hence, why I'm contributing to this book.

I've been on a deep spiritual and conscious personal journey since a very young age, and I came to realise that just because I was never driven by money or material wealth, that there's nothing wrong with me. I've always been of service and impact-driven, so I knew that by making peace with myself and living even more in alignment with my core values, that prosperity would follow.

So often in life, we let others identify what we feel and who we are. We allow them to take our power and our energy, which leaves us depleted, disconnected and empty.

I was a sensitive child who was often sick. While hidden within my inner world, I became fascinated with energy. I was curious about where our life force comes from and how I could become stronger and healthier.

During my childhood, there was a sense of heaviness in my family. My mother was often unwell. She looked sad and not at all joyful. Actually, I can hardly remember her smiling. I wanted to understand why that was and how to help her. My need to connect and play with my mum set me on my path of learning about human behaviour.

I grew up in a communist regime. My perception was that it didn't really allow for a lot of expression and individuality. It was more focused on collective brotherhood and solidarity based on authoritarian leadership. My experience was that people, or at least the ones around me, didn't really thrive. There was a sense of oppression and suppression.

My family and I were secretly going to church, and I remember feeling confused about what I was allowed to be, think and feel. Moreover, I didn't know who it was safe to be, and nothing made much sense. All I wanted was to be happy and free, and it seemed life and freedom came with a lot of written and unwritten rules. I aspired to break free and dreamed about leaving the country, which I later did.

The communist regime was followed by the war, and that took me on an even deeper journey of understanding the suffering around me. I just couldn't comprehend why human beings would ever want to kill each other. What could possibly drive them to do such a thing? People's neighbours and friends they'd known for years, suddenly turned against each other. I wanted to grasp the driving force and power behind it.

I remember thinking that no war is between individuals. It's between the collective forces represented by certain identities, ideologies and values. This idea made me question my own personal ideals, so I went on a search for my humanity and spirituality.

I became passionate about discovering ways to help people end suffering and find their personal truth and power, so they could co-create peace and wellbeing.

My life and work experience made me believe that when people are connected with their innate power, their essence and higher love, they can create a new vibrational reality without wars, violence and destructive behaviour.

How can people get in touch with their core values?

The experience of your life is defined by knowing you're guided by your own true values, while understanding who you are on a deeper level and living your Why.

The thing is, no one goes through life without challenges and adversity. The important question to ask yourself is what you can do and what you can learn when you face them. How do you find the strength to lift your spirits, so you don't give up and fall into depression and anxiety? The key process is to investigate your inner spiritual home, your Why, and to get in touch with your core values that will guide your life in alignment with your true self.

Life isn't easy at times. I don't want to sugar-coat it. We've all experienced pain and suffering, and we're all part of a shared humanity and human experience. We can choose to pretend we're okay, but deep down we know if that's true or not. The opportunity to choose your truth is always yours, and it's always there.

My motto is...
It's never too late to choose love over fear.

When facing challenges and making decisions, ask yourself, *What would love do now?*

What gives your life meaning?

Having clients from all over the world, I can confidently say we all have challenges and feel worn out, but it's the decisions we make during these times that will determine our quality of life, as well as our future.

I always feel privileged to hear someone's life story. I feel honoured that they've trusted me to be their guide from their deepest pain to fulfilment and success, and I don't take that privilege for granted.

To be someone's coach, their guide on the side, and hold their hand on their journey of self-discovery, deep love and fulfilling success, gives meaning to my life. I will do absolutely everything I can to make sure their quality of life improves and their soul shines.

In truth, we're all looking for the same thing, what Brené Brown describes as a 'whole-hearted life'. One of my precious moments is when I heard Brené say, "Vulnerability is the most accurate measurement of courage". This brought so much liberation to me! I'm a huge empath. I feel everything! Understanding the power of vulnerability helped me become a great healer and to connect with others on a deep level.

I gave myself permission to feel and be free. To be real and authentic.

After searching for my true identity and purpose, I came to realise that it's loving and serving others.

"The ability to be vulnerable is not a weakness, it's a strength. You are born courageous and free."

What is energy?

We all have the ability to feel energy. It's a palpable and animated life force. Some days we may be in a state of low energy, and on others, high energy. We can certainly perceive changes in our body just by gauging how we feel. Furthermore, we notice differences in our productivity, our life, our work and relationships, based on our levels of energy.

After working with clients and energy for over twenty years, I've come to understand that even people who've never had experience with energy healing and body work, often describe that they feel low in energy and blocked, or that their energy isn't flowing.

Whether it's work, relationships, health, or just life in general, one of the most common statements I hear is, "I feel stuck". The thing is, your energetic body system can be impacted by certain blocks that will manifest in your physical, emotional, cognitive and energy body.

My area of fascination for the past couple of decades, has been energy, life force and our innate power. I wanted to find out how we could become conscious creators energised from within, so we could live to our fullest potential. What I discovered was that by changing and elevating our energy, the quality of our life changes as well.

"Your energy is your life! Your energy is your best business card."

How can people 'unstuck/unblock' their energy?

Here are four helpful tools to help you unstuck your energy:

1. **Be grounded in your body.**
   Remember to release other people's energy by using your intention. Take a few deep breaths in through the top of your head and down through your body, and then breathe out, allowing this energy to completely exit your body and energy field. Be aware of your feet on the ground, touching the earth.

2. **Be fully embodied in your personal aura space.**
   Each person has an energetic aura. Be aware of your aura boundaries, and inhabit your whole energy field on a daily basis. Visualise it about an arm's length away from your body in all directions. Feel the edges of your aura, stable and strong.

3. **Practice energy hygiene.**
   Use highly vibrational golden energy to purify your mind, body and spirit. Imagine having a golden energy shower coming in through the top of your head and down through your whole energetic body space, with the intention of clearing and releasing the energy that's unproductive and draining.

4. **Reclaim your energy from all people, places, times and events.**
   Do this exercise daily.

   Create an image, and connect with the golden sun. Breathe the golden light into your mind, body and energy field, hold for few seconds, and then gently breathe out. Feel expansion in your energy body.

In summary: On a daily basis, isolate and release from your mind, body and spirit all of the energy, vibrations, thoughts and emotions that are not yours and are not for your divine highest good.

What does it mean to be in a state of flow?

Energy is a constant. It's a natural force that can't be created or destroyed, but can be *altered and transformed*.

When my ten-year-old daughter asks me "Mum, why do people do bad things to other people?", my answer is, "It's always about consciousness and how aware people are of what is happening inside of them".

"The more conscious you are of your feelings and thoughts, the more you become aware of your energy. Once this happens, you can consciously direct your energy, behaviour and actions towards kindness, acceptance, positive creation, connection, love and joy."

Personal and spiritual development, and the study of flow, have become increasingly more popular. When we experience moments of flow, we trust and surrender our life and feel harmonious. We're in a state of receptivity, allowing ourselves to be present and accepting of what is. We realise we can't control the external world, but we have the power to master our internal one.

When there's flow, there's no resistance, no stress or anxiety about the future. We have an embodied experience of being present with an open mind and heart, and deep rhythmic breath. There's a sense of spaciousness in our body, our consciousness and our energy.

"When you're in a state of flow, you no longer feel stuck and closed off to life, opportunities and people."

Just saying out loud, "I no longer need to control my life and force it to happen. It's safe for me to be and let go", will bring you a sense of relief and peace in your energy field.

Letting go of control and trusting life is challenging for many people, but once we choose inner trust and higher guidance, there's no longer a need to force the current of energy into something or someone.

Questions to ask yourself:
- Am I consciously living my life?
- Do I trust myself?

- Do I trust life?
- How am I in the area of self-love?
- Do I feel worthy?
- Do I feel enough?

When you go into avoidance and choose to disconnect from yourself and others, you need to ask yourself why.

> "You're worthy of knowing your love, inner truth and purpose.
> Be your best friend, not your own worst enemy."

How can people move out of victim mode and into empowerment?

People can expend a huge amount of energy on self-sabotage, fear and anxiety. It's the energetic print we learned, but we can also unlearn it. Imagine, instead, having all of that energy to unleash for your conscious life creation.

In my Inner Healer and Inner Leader Activation Program, the emphasis is on emotional, mental and spiritual self-mastery. We're multidimensional human beings who are also highly intelligent. The journey of self-discovery and self-leadership is truly extraordinary.

Inner work and self-exploration can be challenging when we're on our own. But with the right support and guidance system, it can be a rewarding and fulfilling experience.

> "Starting from today, this very moment, start appreciating your life, and honour yourself for all of the challenges you've been through.
>
> You're here now and your life is precious."

Regardless of our careers and different life experiences, we're all leaders and impact-makers in one form or another. Life happens from the inside out, not the other way around. My aspiration is to help people move out from their victim mentality and into leadership, empowerment and high energy, in order to fulfil their purpose of life creation.

When I was introduced to Stedman Graham, American educator, businessmen, author and Oprah's partner, his work and wisdom were so inspiring to me. That very moment, I decided to commit to writing a book. Words from his speech stayed with me. He said, "To know yourself is the first and most important step in pursuing your dreams and goals".

"To lead others, first you must know how to lead yourself."

The beauty of self-discovery is that the more we're at home within ourselves, and the more energy and love we have for our very own existence, we come to realise that our personal development isn't just for us, but the whole world. When we become aware of who we are and our life force, we're empowered and present in the flow of our life, and the distortion and abuse of power will change.

How can people make a difference in the world?

We can all make a difference by moving from I-consciousness into We-consciousness. By caring for others and realising we're all part of the same humanity, and that we're all interconnected, we begin to make contributions towards the improvement of our energy and the planet.

Once we realign our own selves, and connect to our energy, our life force and innate power, we'll understand that we all have the ability to make a difference in our lives and the lives of others.

How can people become conscious and aware of their energy?

1. **Breathe deeply**
    Be conscious of your breath. What does your breathing feel like? Is it rapid and shallow, or deep?

2. **Be present**
    Go inward, and check in with yourself. How do you feel physically, mentally and emotionally?

▶ Check in with your mind

- What is your mind doing?
- Understand that you are not your mind, and you are not what you think. Your thoughts are forms of energy and vibration.
- Be aware of your thoughts and stories in your head. What is true? What are you choosing to think about?

▶ Check in with your feelings

- How are you feeling?
- Understand that you are not your emotions. Witness them, but don't identify yourself with them.
- Emotions are energy in motion. Let them move through your body. Don't hold onto them. Feel them, and let them go.

▶ Check in with your body

- How does your body feel?
- Is there any pain or discomfort? If so, locate where it is, and send love to that part of your body.
- Move your body regularly.

▶ Connect with, and be aware of your energy

- What happens to your energy and your energy field when you do certain actions?

- What about when you're around certain people? Is your energy expanding or contracting?
- Do you feel drained, depleted, inspired or uplifted?

Why is meditation so important?

Most people say "Sleep on it", and I always say, "Meditate on it".

From my experience, meditation is one of the best ways to get to know yourself on a deeper, more intimate level.

Prayer is action outwards, and meditation is action inwards.

I see prayer as talking to God, Source, Universal Energy, or however you choose to refer to it, that's in alignment with your belief system, and meditation as listening to God, creation or energy inside of your being.

A healing journey of self-discovery is exciting and causes you to realise that life can transform in a heartbeat.

Meditation and energy work changed my life. During my childhood, I was ill and allergic to so many things, and at times had difficulty breathing. It wasn't much fun being unwell and missing out on playing with my friends.

I was prescribed many different medications and became so tired of blood tests and visits to doctors and hospitals.

One day I came home, and I said to myself, *"Enough is enough". I'm not getting better, and I don't want to spend my life being sick. There must be another way!*

I decided to change my ways by trying something different. As the famous quote goes, "Insanity is doing the same thing over and over again, expecting different results". So when I was twelve-years-old, I decided to stop taking all of my medication and look for alternative ways to heal.

As I've mentioned before, I was fascinated with what gives us energy to live and breathe. My interest in the metaphysical started early in life. I was going to church all the time to find out about my higher power, love, truth and God.

Somehow, I also had a natural ability to transcend, and I'd lose myself for hours and hours being in nature and meditating. I felt like I was finding my happiness. I enjoyed my inner world, even though my outer world wasn't the easiest place to be.

Years went by, and at the age of twenty-two, I had just graduated university and became a primary school teacher, when I was introduced to Reiki. I was then taken on a journey all the way to a Master level.

For years, I spent weekends in Reiki courses, meditation and channelling. I absolutely loved it. Interestingly, I went from someone who was sick all the time, to someone who no longer took any painkillers or medications, and my body got well. My spirit was happy!

I felt safe knowing my internal guidance system and inner healer would always steer me in the right direction. My intuition brought me to Australia to study for a Master of International Relations, so I could change the world. Or so I thought! I came to realise that my calling was to work with energy, consciousness and leadership. People's happiness had always mattered to me.

My spiritual quest brought me to India, where I experienced divine energy and the love of a divine mother. It felt like coming home. My daughter and I spent a lot of time in Peedam, and I became acquainted with so many amazing people and charitable projects.

It was there my spiritual teacher gave me my new mantra, which became my guiding principle: *Om Namo Narayani*. It means, 'I surrender to the divine'. The practice of chanting is truly transformational. When I work with clients, especially if they have a 'busy monkey mind', I give them a personal mantra.

When people come to me and say, "I can't meditate!" it's often because they think their mind needs to stop, and they believe they need to do it forcefully.

However, this is not the case. The simple practice of meditation only requires you to sit comfortably while observing what your mind is doing and how your body is feeling. You can start with five or ten minutes a day. There's no need to force anything. Just be a witness to your meditative practice, and allow divine energy to flow through you.

The key is to be consistent and not resist painful feelings, because what we resist, persists.

When I work with clients, I help them release any blockages that prevent them from being able to meditate and connect deeper with their essence and stillness of their being.

By practising your mantra and meditation, your mind will begin to understand that it's a tool in service to your purpose and the creation of a meaningful and fulfilling life.

You'll be more conscious of what you feed your mind and if it's adding value to your life and purpose. Once you realise you're a divine being, you naturally make healthier and more loving choices.

How can people become aware of their higher needs?

According to Abraham Maslow and his hierarchy of needs, self-actualisation is the highest goal of our lives. I don't entirely agree with his theory, which feels somewhat linear to me. Once you enter the world of metaphysical energy and vibration, you realise time and life aren't necessarily linear.

Maslow's theory starts with fulfilling our basic needs for food and shelter before we can climb the ladder to meet our higher ones. While it does seem that western culture can be focused on more basic material needs, it doesn't necessarily mean people are linearly getting to their self-actualisation and fulfilment. Life is like a living, breathing organism, and it happens in the here and now. If we're not present, embodied and connected, then how can we have the full life experience?

Throughout my life journey and work, I can say that we no longer need years of therapy and a linear approach to life, healing and fulfilment. Conscious living, and creating your life consciously, will set you on a fulfilling path. Eckhart Tolle describes how some people identify with their thinking mind and the movement of thoughts. It reacts to everything that happens around them, and the narrative it creates depends upon how a person's mind is conditioned due to past experiences. Without awareness, they can only identify with the narrative their mind has constructed.

You've probably heard people say, "I'm tired of thinking". What you need is to have a masterful mind that doesn't drain you and your energy with constant activity.

"Awareness is the key!"

When you face challenges, your mind doesn't just look into what's happening now. It looks into data from the past and projects to the future. In accordance with this theory, it will create your reality. Once you become aware of what your mind is doing, you can be present and alter the experience of your current reality.

What are the essential steps to mastering the mind?

Here are the five essential steps to mastering your mind:

1. **Be present**
   Consciously breathe and awaken to the present moment.
2. **Be aware**
   Be aware of what your mind is creating and what you're thinking.
3. **Observe**
   Don't identify yourself with your mind. Be an observer.
4. **Meditate**
   Meditate daily.
5. **Practise gratitude**
   Give thanks.

Daily practise: Presence in the Now. Breathing for calm composure, renewed energy and focus.

Breathe in through your nose and into your belly for a mental count of four, hold and then breathe out through your nose for a count of eight. When you first begin, repeat three times, and then with practise, increase to two-three minutes.

When you come to your senses, identify what you can hear, see and smell.

Finish with *Om Namo Narayani* (I surrender to the divine).

How can people achieve fulfilment and joy?

Let your energy be your best business card.

Our energetic presence and vibration are more important than our words.

When I came across Dr Milton Erickson and his work around the power of the conscious and unconscious mind, I was fascinated with the study of rapport. He realised that when human beings get in rapport, they begin to mirror each other.

I observed this theory from the point of energy and vibration and the Law of Attraction. I became captivated with watching people's energy when they communicated with each other and what happened within their energy field. What I came to understand was that our energy and vibration will speak for us before we even attempt to connect and verbalise.

I've seen so many people who've tried for years to make successful alterations in their life. They've attended courses and worked on their mindset. They'd been told to take massive action, and very often by the time they came to see me, they were tired and depleted, experiencing heartaches and all sorts of dissatisfaction and pain. Even those who often achieved so much in their lives still weren't fulfilled. They had no energy to enjoy their life.

The journey to fulfilment and true success starts from the inside out. Inner awareness and connection with the core of your being is essential for a meaningful and happy life. Working together, we can combine spiritual and energy principles in all areas. Your life experience is directly connected to, and is a reflection of your energy. To make long-lasting changes in your life, an identity and energy shift is vital.

"You realise you are a powerful, sovereign being on a mission!"

What is the power of giving?

I believe that the power of giving is something inside of us that is greater than ourselves.

Regardless of our background and differences in beliefs, we can agree that we all share the same sky and sun, and have the experience of shared humanity. There's something amazing that happens inside of us when we feel we've helped another human being.

The power of giving is truly transformational, and we all have something to give. When we experience another person receiving our love, kindness, compassion and financial help, it's the most fulfilling and rewarding experience we can have.

The secret to a meaningful and fulfilling life, is giving.
You can instantaneously revive your life and energy by being of service and bringing joy to others.

Life is a miracle, and feeling connected to a higher love, to your true self, brings you wholeness, new energy and a new reality, where life creation happens from your being, your inner self.

You realise that you're powered from within and inseparable from higher love and life force energy.

Now is the perfect time to become empowered and equipped to elevate your energy. Activate your inner healer and leader, so you can create a life that's in alignment with who you are and what you value the most. Allow your life to become a more effortless, fulfilling experience with the joy of living and giving.

"Fulfilment comes from your true essence. Live your life aligned with the energy of your soul, and know that you're powered from within to love and be loved."

In loving service and gratitude,
Marina Rei

To discover more about how Marina can help you *Elevate Your Energy*, simply visit www.elevatebooks.com/energy

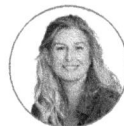

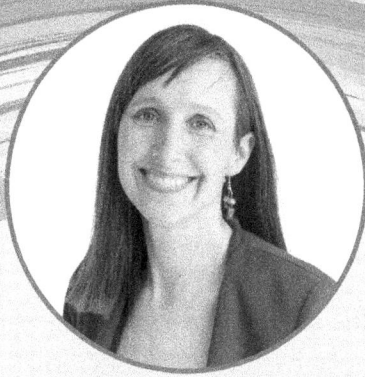

Robyn Reynolds
Empowering Energy

Robyn Reynolds is a teacher, writer, researcher, presenter and natural therapist, who helps people get in sync with their inner self and live a more intuitive life.

Robyn's interest in assisting people with their unique individual development led her to the study of kinesiology, which she believes is the perfect bridge between her scientific knowledge and her desire to help people direct their own learning and healing.

Through her coaching and kinesiology businesses, Robyn provides insight, highly effective techniques and programs for fast change.

Robyn is passionate about guiding her clients to identify what they really want and having them clear their energetic blockages, so they can make the small changes that create a huge, positive knock-on effect.

Robyn Reynolds

Empowering Energy

What is your biggest life lesson?

No matter what others think, it's my own judgement that matters the most. I need to live up to my own personal standards. Nobody knows exactly what others are basing their judgments on anyway, so I made the decision to be my own judge and to be kind to myself in the process.

This was a big lesson for me to learn. In the past, I was always trying to please others. As a child, I tried living according to what other people thought was right or important. I spent time imagining I was somebody else, exploring the personas and perspectives of many of those around me. It wasn't done with judgement, or even fun, as such. Just pure curiosity and a deep thirst for information.

This was part of how I learned about myself through the people around me. But it was also an avoidance of getting to know myself, because I was scared to disagree with anyone, in case I would offend. I wanted to get things right by other people's standards and began to ignore my own ideas.

This led to a feeling that I never had enough energy to do what I really wanted, and I often felt tired and unmotivated. I had to push myself to complete my studies, while constantly snacking during lectures to stay awake and ingested many coffees and energy drinks to try and get more energy. I would get stuck 'all in my head' while feeling physically unable to move or connect to my emotional side.

In the long run, my physical health suffered. I'd been ignoring chronic gut pains, I had frequent colds that would last for weeks on end, and many aches, pains and postural issues that made walking barefoot or sitting on the ground a chore. This wasn't right, but I trooped on as I thought that's what I was supposed to do.

When I started my career as a biomedical engineer, working to service and repair medical equipment, I found it interesting but not fulfilling. After changing jobs three times in two years, I took time out to travel the world. I learned a lot about myself and developed many amazing new perspectives.

Soon after returning, my physical health problems caught up with me. I had a cold I just couldn't kick. I was exhausted, unable to work and facing chronic fatigue in my twenties. Then a downhill skiing accident made sure I stayed put and accept that I had to slow down and put some serious effort into figuring out my health and my life.

What is the one message you wish to share with the world?

That we're all connected, and our universe is non-linear and dynamic. It ebbs and flows, rather than always following a predictable, linear course. In nature there are many patterns that exist on multiple levels, such as the shape of a leaf being like the overall shape of the tree. These repeated patterns of similarity are referred to as 'fractals'.

Learning this from the mathematics I studied at university inspired me to explore the concept that it's possible to map our physical body to the earth and observe where the fractal similarities are. For example, if you scrutinise an imaging of our lungs, you'll notice they look like trees, and trees are effectively the lungs of the earth.

Our DNA holds patterns that can manifest in our physical body, and it is possible to detect potential issues before they turn into a problem. This knowledge has enabled me to develop ways of working with others to easily identify the new desired pattern and effectively install it in an intentional way, to bring about optimal health and wellness.

These insights show our significance and power to influence, or be influenced, because we're all part of this shared space. When we're living our best lives and making the most of being here in physical form during this lifetime, we can use these natural laws of physics to our advantage. Just as our world is dynamically changing around us, we, too, must be able to flex and change, which is best done from a sturdy base.

Know who you are intricately. Rather than trying to merely calculate your next move based on a formula with all the known inputs, be open to the information that is yet to be defined. Understand yourself and your own boundaries, but be open to what can initially seem strange or irritating, as this can be the key to what you need to know or work on next.

It's good to understand what's going on and to keep that childhood curiosity of always asking why. It's also necessary to be comfortable with the mystery that remains for questions that can't be answered yet. You can theorise and tune into the possibilities.

In order to receive the knowledge, you need to approach a situation with fresh eyes and tap into your innate knowledge and intuition, that of the ancients through place, history or imaginings. Allow all of this to guide your research. Be prepared to set aside what you already know and be in a place of inquisitive wonder.

Challenges to your existing view of the world can cause conflicts, especially when you want to feel smart. But if you truly desire to change for the better, it's often necessary to set previous judgements aside and allow yourself to be vulnerable. Some of your thoughts and beliefs are from a collective consciousness or the messages society's influencers are offering.

I believe we have many more senses than merely sight, hearing, taste, touch and smell. We are, in fact, electrical and magnetic beings. There's so much we still don't understand about our electromagnetic nature and how it affects those around us. And the more knowledge we acquire, the more we realise we have a lot to learn. This is why it's so vital to be in tune with our own inner messages and to honour the expression of our intuitive selves.

Have you had any aha moments that changed everything for you?

Wow, yes, I have. The big one that resonates throughout my life came to me in an instant at some point in my mid-twenties. It was the culmination of much philosophical thought after I completed my degrees in science and engineering. I was supposed to know everything now, right? But I just had more questions.

In learning much about how the world works through these physical sciences, including the invisible mechanics of electronics, it was clear to me that we don't know everything yet. Our science is highly valued and useful for creating new technologies, but it's also evolving. One new discovery can have an impact on what we thought was set in stone.

Instead of fearing that everything could suddenly come crumbling down, I became curious about this mystery. At first, I was dumbfounded by the concept that no one knows everything and probably never will. But then I realised it's because the deeper we go, the more opportunity there is for greater understanding. This idea has led me to research and put information from different disciplines together to explore the possibilities of what's going on. It's made me appreciate that we don't need to know everything to make progress, especially when it comes to healing and living in a good energy space.

It was clear to me from the mathematical models for the cutting-edge physics of the time, that due to the non-linear nature of things, a carefully placed small change can make a world of difference under the right circumstances. This is referred to as the Butterfly Effect and is typically discussed in relation to weather systems, but can also apply to many other systems as well. I regularly observe this effect at play during sessions with clients.

I also realised how this information applied to me spiritually. Though I wasn't sure if I believed there was anything out there or not, I understood that, for example, nobody knows scientifically if a God exists or if there's anything more. At that time, nobody knew if the universe was expanding or contracting, either. I came to the conclusion that it was purely my choice to believe what I wanted. I weighed up the pros and cons to decide whether it was better for me to believe there's something out there that we're connected to, or to remain unaware. For me, the answer came easily. I choose to believe, which I trusted would give me the most positive framework for my life and get me comfortable with the mystery.

What decisions have made a difference in your life?

The big one was my decision to take responsibility for my health. It meant I had to accept that I could no longer be a victim. This was a huge shift for me and took some time to unpack.

Certain parts of my journey felt like one step forward, two steps back, but it was vital to reclaiming my energy and tapping into an abundant source. I think prior to that epiphany, I was getting a lot of secondary gain from "poor me" whenever bad things "happened" to me. I had to rebuild my relationship with myself and learn how to interact with others in a totally different way from what I was used to. It's funny that I took this approach, because I so desperately needed my health to improve, and it actually wound up flowing into all areas of my life in such an empowering way.

Health is often a reflection of what's going on in other aspects of your life, so it makes a lot of sense. Poor health can be viewed as a message that you have something out of balance and gives you the guidance you need to recalibrate.

In my sessions, I help clients decipher the clues and use them to improve their overall situation. When teaching, I encourage people to be in charge of their own learning. I love that I've created a life where I now get to share this empowerment with others. I'm on a mission to motivate and facilitate self-responsibility in all areas of life, so we can live in communities with a responsible, free lifestyle. In other words, a state of interdependence, a word coined by Stephen Covey in *The 7 Habits of Highly Effective People*.

What do you think is the biggest problem people face?

That they give their power to others instead of taking responsibility for their health, education and life in general. They survive by becoming the victim instead of making empowering decisions that help them thrive. It's an easy trap to fall into, and I'm certainly still susceptible to this at times.

Now, just to be clear, I'm not saying bad things don't happen, that they're the fault of the victim or even that there's always a meaning. This can be as fruitless an approach as dwelling on the past, going over and over it and re-energising it as a badge of honour, when it's just a source of pain or negativity. No, this is about shifting the focus to learning, gaining insight and being inspired to help others, or turning it into a positive force in some way.

What's the best way to help them with this problem?

Holding the space and helping them understand and shift their perspective. If it's all someone else's fault, then who is controlling them? Who gets the most out of them deciding to change things for the better?

You need to realise and be in awe of your own power to manage all that you can control. There's always something you can do. A new framework or perspective is required. It's your life you're living. Start from this moment, and accept that it might take a while to process everything. You're in charge, and you're allowed to seek help, too. Put together a team to let you know what your options are from their area of expertise, and then consider your own information, circumstances and consequences. You're the one who knows the most about you.

How did you become interested in changing careers and helping others instead of servicing medical equipment?

I knew I wanted to help others after all the support I received in rebuilding my own health. I'm a people person at heart, but a contributing factor to my fatigue and lack of motivation was that I was spending my workdays alone with machines. Needless to say, the conversations were all a little one-sided. I wanted to take what I learned from my hospital work and education, and integrate it into how I could help others improve their own lives.

So began my dream of becoming a health practitioner. But a practitioner of what? Or was there some other way?

I was intrigued by quantum physics and the potential to tap into our body's own innate healing powers. I learned about using specific energetic frequencies to detect health issues and how they could also be used to help the body heal. I was inspired by my naturopath, who'd coached me through my recovery, but this would take another four years of study.

I considered degrees in psychology and social work. I took short courses in meditation, reiki, psychology, life writing, flower essences and counselling. I visited a number of places that were offering courses in natural therapies and looked into a variety of short courses and workshops. Getting regular chiropractic adjustments had helped me, so maybe I could start with learning massage?

Feeling overwhelmed, I knew I needed to work with my existing strengths. Figuring out how things work, and sharing this information with others, had always come naturally for me. I'd often tutored mathematics and volunteered at a school to help out in maths classes. Everything lined up in a manner that allowed me to complete my teaching qualifications within the year, and I started teaching work soon after.

While working as a school teacher, I spent some time learning about kinesiology and the pathways to study it that would allow me to continue teaching. This is what ticked all the boxes for me and seemed the most likely to bring my existing knowledge about energy systems into practice. I was also excited about how kinesiology could help with learning difficulties, as well as health and any goal you might like to set for yourself.

What courses have you taken that enabled you to start your own business?

My kinesiology diploma not only enabled me to start my business, but has helped me with my life in every way. I came to know my true needs and tune in to my own intuition, which has been a total game changer. I think in the past I'd been rejecting a whole lot of inner messages and hence was rejecting a part of myself. Not good.

I'd also completed a course in small business management, which quickly gave me confidence with bookkeeping and following the rules and requirements for running a business. This meant I didn't have to muddle along or try to work it all out myself. I was also connected with a mentor, and the wealth of insight they provided, both personally and business-wise, was amazingly insightful and inspiring.

Completing my certification in results coaching and other personal and business development courses, has enabled me to take my work to a whole other level over the past few years. I'm able to have a more holistic approach, working with clients virtually with more flexibility and efficiency.

What is your most inspiring client story?

I'm always amazed how the work I do can facilitate rapid change in people's physical health. It's nice to see, as they're often more tangible and measurable than the mental, emotional or spiritual changes.

I recall one of my clients was able to boost a struggling system in their body from fifty or sixty percent functionality, before briefly jumping up to one-hundred percent, and then levelling out at around eighty percent thereafter. Their results amazed their specialists, and they were able to skip their planned surgery.

The people I work with are continually inspiring me. I'm always open to all possibilities, as I appreciate that I never know their full story. It really is up to them as to what they're capable of achieving. What inspires me the most is witnessing people making the conscious connections with what they need to do and finding the synchronicity that makes life exciting and easy for them to achieve what they want.

I'm also fascinated when clients tell me that other people in their lives have changed and are interacting with them differently. I assume this is subconscious, where the other person is picking up on their energy. They say that we rise to the expectations of others. From what I can see, that's generally true in the case of interpersonal interactions, even when the expectations are felt within the client and not necessarily communicated directly to those around them. This inspires me to research more about how our own electromagnetic fields interact with other people's.

What do you think is your life purpose?

Helping others be truly present and honest with themselves, so they can see all of their options and live more intuitive lives. I want to activate the necessary changes in people that will awaken them to their fullest potential and empower them to operate from a high-vibrational state, so they can live purposeful lives and inspire others.

It's easy to get stuck endlessly studying science and rationalising everything mentally, or to go all emotional, being reactive, stubborn or aloof. Getting these aspects integrated, and being able to utilise all of your senses instead of just the obvious ones, gets you more in line with what your life purpose really is. If you're genuinely connected to yourself and coming from a place of love and care for yourself and others, the world could be full of synchronous symphonies, as your interconnections play out more harmoniously. Facilitating and educating people about this transformational healing process is what I am dedicated to.

Why do you think people are working in a job they dislike?

There are a lots of good excuses people tell themselves, whether it's to meet their financial responsibilities, to retain their sense of identity, not wanting to waste what they've invested in training, a perceived lack of other options or just not wanting to make the effort to change. It's easy to get stuck, as so much time spent in an environment you don't like can wear you down and affect your motivation, as well as your mental and physical health.

There can often be unconscious and energetic reasons, too. One of the things I find most exciting when coaching clients is when we work on shifting the energy first, new career opportunities are able to appear or be recognised. The transition can be easy and practical, without negative impacts on their lifestyle.

Another factor to consider for people not liking their job is the aspects they focus on. What we focus on and spend more time thinking about expands in our consciousness. Too much focus on the negative is possible to work on as well. Removing negative beliefs and changing them for yourself, creates new attitudes and perspectives that affect the way you interact with the various aspects of the role you play in your own life and with those around you. A focus on what you're grateful for can improve your feelings towards it, whether you love it, dislike it or outright find it abhorrent.

How can people overcome fear?

First, recognise exactly what you're being fearful of. Then consider if it were to happen what the worst-case scenario would be, but don't dwell on it. Be fully honest with yourself. This removes uncertainty and can be enough to dispel the fear.

Often the next step is to identify what skills you would need to best deal with the situation causing you fear. You might decide to upskill or fill in the gaps of your knowledge. The clarity and certainty help to remove it. Your subconscious can get curious and want to explore your fears if you don't consciously face them. Figure out what you need to do.

Clearing stress patterns caused by anxiety and past trauma, reduces the triggering of our stress responses. Less time spent in fight/flight/

freeze mode increases your opportunity of imagining a positive alternative to your fear, so you project that energy instead. This puts the fear in its place and shuts off the negativity you could otherwise attract into your life.

How can someone find their life purpose?

Get to know your likes and dislikes, and then choose a purpose that's aligned with it. What excites you? Use it as a guide. Do activities that connect you deeply to yourself, and allow your intuition to guide you. Maybe you have more than one potential life purpose to live out or a whole list of options to choose from. You can also try doing something that moves you closer to your purpose, even if you're not sure what that is or what it will become once you get there.

What are you passionate about?

I'm passionate about helping people align to the energy of what they want. Once the pattern is there energetically, the rest is much easier to achieve. Changes in physical, mental and emotional states can seem automatic when you're energetically aligned to your intended outcome. This concept can be applied to health, learning, wellness, sport and any goals you want to achieve.

Why are goals important?

Goals help you live your life on purpose, rather than being at the whim of circumstance. It's a vital part of taking full responsibility for yourself. Goals can be the key to protecting and maintaining the lifestyle you love or getting you to take active steps towards achieving it.

Wouldn't it be wonderful if you could just stop time and put all of your perfect systems in place, and then never have to do it again? But this is not reality. Change is a certainty. Having goals shapes your life in the direction you want it to, instead of being subject to other people's intentions.

What is the best way to set and achieve goals?

I think this can vary depending on the individual. In our sessions, I help people find a method that can become part of a routine they look forward to.

The way I work with clients when they're not clear on their goal, is that we take their problem, or what's frustrating them, and flip it to the positive. It then becomes a positive affirmation, which allows us to explore the way it sits with them and to clear any energetic clutter, such as conflicts or blockages. We're basically creating and putting the new thought or belief in place to make it easy for the changes to happen.

Next, we get specific with the details of the goal, when they aim to achieve it, and how to know when they've achieved it. We then integrate it with the vision they have of themselves for their future, and look at what steps are involved, before breaking them down to appropriately sized tasks. Going from having an issue they can't solve to achieving their goals, encourages gratitude for the lessons learned.

How can people be happier?

Be organised, be present, practice gratitude and clear past traumas, big and small. Learn lessons from everyday life experiences. Study history and humanity. Delve deeply into who you really are. Bravely embrace all sides of what you may discover about yourself. Be your own judge, and evolve to be the you that you choose to be.

Open yourself up to possibilities. For me, this concept appeared through physics and maths. It's crazy how much we don't know, but when you look closely enough at the models, you will see there's space for limitless possibility that are sometimes prompted by the smallest changes. Get an idea of the bigger picture, and know what you want. Take it one step at a time. Schedule fun time and downtime.

How can people be healthier?

If I had to narrow it down to one sentence, I'd say, "Be more intuitive". Allow your physical, emotional and mental components to align, and accept that there are energetic and spiritual components at play, whether you're conscious of them or not. Approach your health with a curiosity to learn. Be ready to listen to the messages and metaphors your physiology is providing for you.

Ask yourself questions like, "What area can I improve next?" It may be time to add, delete or modify some of the foods you're consuming or tidy up your house. Your outer world reflects your inner one, and you can use this in either direction to get healthier. Look around you for the clues:

- Have I allowed my creative spaces to become cluttered?
- Why is my body having an imbalance?
- What is it telling me I do or don't need?

Answering these questions can sometimes be enough for you to have a revelation that clears the disempowering energy. Then the next step becomes a more meaningful, health-promoting activity that replaces emotionally damaging motivators such as guilt, stress and negative self-talk. I have some great processes I use with clients to facilitate this inner work.

Be dynamic in your approach, and continue making changes to balance things out. There's no one-size-fits-all approach. Be grateful for your health, and take a proactive role in finding what's best for you at that time. The support of a coach, your own knowledge and research, and any other experts you think might help, can provide fresh eyes and insight.

Why is health important?

Because it provides an overall imprint for your lifestyle. When you feel good, you do your best and achieve what you want in life. Being proactive with your health leads you to healthy relationships and activism, as you share your spaces with others. Be assertive about your health needs, not only for yourself, but to make a statement as a role model for others to do the same. This contributes to good energy and health for our planet.

Why do you think so many people are overwhelmed and unhappy?

An important factor here that's often overlooked, is that we can easily take on the patterns of what's going on around us without realising it. Our environment is polluted in ways we can clearly notice but also in ways that are invisible and difficult to consciously detect. This can be dangerous, as it sets us up for synchronising to a sad and overwhelmed system. It helps to be intentional in what we choose to align our energies with, and to realise that others will reflect the energetic patterns that we exude.

This makes me think of Masaru Emoto and his book *The Hidden Messages in Water*. Masaru took photographs of water crystals under many conditions and discovered that water has the ability to copy information. The water crystals that formed were beautiful, symmetrical and complete when they were exposed to the words *love and gratitude* but were just the opposite when words such as *you fool* were directed at them instead.

This is relevant to us, because our bodies are made up of a great deal of water. So just as the water crystals reacted to the positive and negative words, it's logical to think that the water in our bodies would be affected similarly. This means that if you're telling yourself off all day for things you forgot or that didn't go as planned, it has a negative effect, as opposed to when you're being loving and appreciating yourself.

What are the best ways people can find energy?

They need to realise it's within them already, and they just need to free it up to make it available. Quality counts over quantity. An example to consider is your sleep and restorative energy. Screen time and artificial lighting has been shown to increase our wake-up hormone, cortisol, which in turn lowers melatonin, our sleep hormone. Poor-quality sleep habits lead to energy depletion during the day. By reducing your exposure to bright lights in the evening, and avoiding screen time for a few hours before bed, you can help yourself sleep better and free up more energy for the daytime.

Clear what's unnecessary and get to know and understand who you are. Being honest with yourself will help you to stop collecting emotional baggage. It's all about the energy. It's necessary to detox and clear clutter not just physically, but mentally, emotionally and spiritually as well. This enables your system to bring itself into balance.

What I find fascinating is that taking action in one area has an effect on other aspects, as your body is a whole system made up of all parts working as a team. It's the same for other systems. There are some things you can't change, so you may need to work indirectly and enable your body to balance out internally. It's the bucket analogy where there's only so much stress that can fit in it, and once it's overflowing, you have a problem.

Biofeedback methods can be a game changer in taking the guesswork out of what you can do to make more room in your bucket. It's especially helpful if the source of your suffering is a mystery, and you don't have a sense of what to prioritise.

In the study of electronics, we bring the invisible into view with schematic diagrams to represent the electric circuits. They include their individual components, the pathways that the electricity will flow through and how it interconnects with other parts within a bigger system.

Similarly, modern and ancient systems of representing our own energy systems also exist. It's empowering to learn about the various energy systems in and around the body, and how to work with these. For example, you can use visualisation to clear and energise your energy centres, energy pathways and energetic connections. These techniques are an empowering key to finding and cultivating access to your energy.

If you were speaking to your younger self, what advice would you give?

You don't need to have a reason to like something. It can be a feeling in your body, or a sensation you may not be able to justify or put into words. You can try new things and expand your identity along the way. You're the person you're stuck with for the rest of your life, so you're the number one person you need to please. Become friends with your emotions. By caring about yourself first, you will be able to know your own highest values and have more good energy to share with others.

Get excited about your future, and nurture it. This includes enjoying the process of building your amazing future, not just pressuring yourself to get it one-hundred-percent perfect right now. It's okay if you make mistakes and change your mind. Play the long game, as it's all a process to experience, rather than just another chore to tick off your to-do list. Right now, be who you want to be in the future, or at least start taking actions that move you in that direction. Stop blocking your intuition, clear your energetic clutter and get in sync with the mystery and magic of life.

"We shall not cease from exploration
And the end of all our exploring
Will be to arrive where we started
And know the place for the first time."
~ *T.S. Eliot, Four Quartets*

To discover more about how Robyn can help you *Elevate Your Energy*, simply visit www.elevatebooks.com/energy

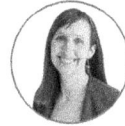

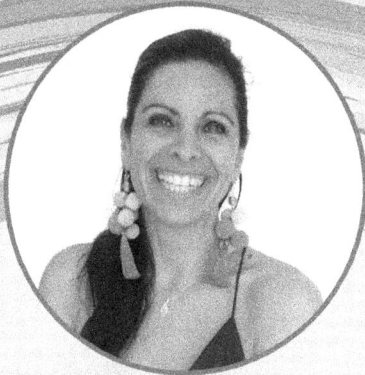

Veronica Galipo

The Power of Words

Veronica Galipo is a certified life coach and practitioner of hypnotherapy, who guides women towards stepping safely into appreciating and embracing themselves, so they can be their own soul-fulfilling best friend.

Through her own personal discovery and healing, Veronica has entwined a mindful and spiritual approach that's reflected in her coaching, soul-lifting techniques and writing. She creates a space where her clients can gain clarity and the truth about themselves, leading them to feel more in tune with their mind and body.

Veronica's greatest gift is how she encourages each individual to reach a place where they live their own unique path, awakening them to a fulfilled, exciting life journey, all because they matter.

Veronica Galipo

The Power of Words

What is your biggest life lesson?

My lesson is to live by my inner real truth.

Sadly, while growing up, this idea was not shared, encouraged or shown to me. I feel I was experiencing a life where you should please and oblige others. I was to fit in, keep the peace, and say and think about what works best for others, rather than standing by myself and sharing my voice.

It took me until my forties to realise that not showing up as my authentic self was depriving my soul and the world of someone living self-assured with inner bliss. When I finally tipped my pinkie toe into the notion that I counted, my purpose began to fall into line, and the golden thread of my soul lit up enough to be seen.

I would love to seep the thought into every small child's heart and mind that their true soul matters. That it's worth looking inside and searching for who they really are, without any layers of other people's stories, beliefs or pictures.

This is why I'm so passionate about the energy and power behind words.

If you were speaking to your younger self, what advice would you give?

This is an exciting question, mainly because I would enjoy this conversation very much, as I do this now with my near-teenage boys.

The main thing I would want to whisper, or actually shout from the rooftops, is, "You're doing fantastic! You're worthy of greatness and love. You are an inspiration, and it's safe to be you".

Always be open to change, and embrace all experiences.

Welcome anything in life that comes your way, even if it looks bad, and know that you can count on the power of your self-consoling and self-assurance to gain wonder from it all.

Look in the mirror, and take in the unique miracle of yourself.

No one else is the combined essence of you, and you have a right to embrace your one life, including all that comes with it and all you can create.

Know that you have a great mind and an immense body power waiting for you to tap into. Use them to create the life that's so ready for you to make your own.

Take note of the power around every story you shape in your mind. Every word or phrase you say about yourself. Because these small clusters of letters you see and think of as 'just words' have incredible energy around them, so much so, that you become what is said and how you describe yourself.

What is the one message you wish to share with the world?

This powerful learning I've been blessed to receive and continue to stand by, is about the power within, especially around conversations with ourselves and how we see and treat ourselves.

Through my studies, self-exploration and development, I've found that when you change what you say and think, you change your feelings, beliefs and interpretations.

This conscious awareness of how we speak to or about ourselves and others, and how we treat ourselves, is a direct reflection of the vibrations that emanate from where our soul sits. This can be reflected in our bodies, mainly through our nervous system. If the vibration is negative, it can create stresses, health issues and illnesses, as well as mental and physical diseases.

I was fortunate to have realised this from my coaching courses, learnings, mentors, clients and practices.

I was totally a different person most of my life, until the last three years. I would always describe my identity as someone struggling with migraines, digestion issues and body aches and pains, who never slept and had low self-esteem. In essence, I had a weak inner belief.

I remember repeating, "I'm just one of those people who doesn't sleep", and "I wake up with a headache every day" as if this was normal. I was shy, with no self-expression or freedom to voice what I believed, and sadly, no self-love whatsoever.

Incredibly, I now have a strong identity of being an empowered, vital woman who lives deeply and with ease, and has a whole lot of self-loving energy. I protect my self from negative words, knowing I have the powerful ability to alter them, so they lift me instead.

The power and energy behind our words and thoughts are life creators and changers. This awareness around self-talk and self-encouragement empowers us, and our whole system can benefit.

From day-to-day living, to goal-setting and endeavouring to reach new heights, hiccups can arise, so it's natural to be on a certain path before deciding you don't want to continue. This is especially true when you hang onto old pictures of yourself, such as the belief that you can't achieve success or cope when there are challenges. This manifests as procrastination and distracting yourself, which steers you further away from completion and more towards feelings of disappointment.

Try taking a conscious moment to converse with yourself. Remind yourself of the changes and successes in your past and how you survived them. Take your time, and use words of encouragement. By acknowledging the small, yet quality steps you've taken to improve your life, your mindset will shift, and you'll have the strength to continue on your path.

This self-reassurance, kindness and care will cause many aspects of your life to work for you, rather than against you.

Self- rewarding contemplation is known to tap directly into your brain, creating an amazing ability to achieve and complete tasks. By changing your thinking and speaking from a place of worth, anything is possible. It impacts you and the people around you. The power is all in your hands. Or in this case, your words.

How to Live - YOU?

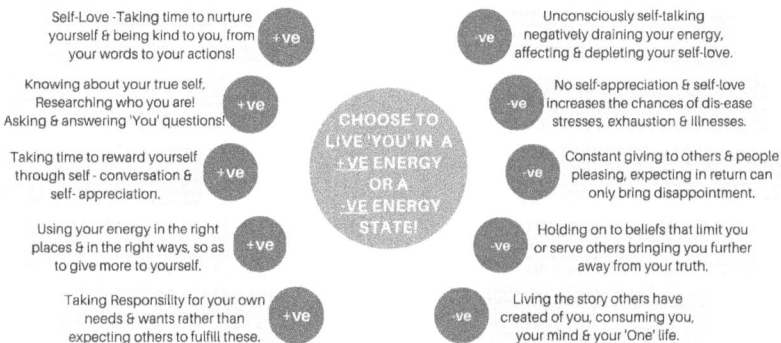

Self-Love -Taking time to nurture yourself & being kind to you, from your words to your actions! **+ve**

Knowing about your true self. Researching who you are! Asking & answering 'You' questions! **+ve**

Taking time to reward yourself through self - conversation & self- appreciation. **+ve**

Using your energy in the right places & in the right ways, so as to give more to yourself. **+ve**

Taking Responsibility for your own needs & wants rather than expecting others to fulfill these. **+ve**

CHOOSE TO LIVE 'YOU' IN A +VE ENERGY OR A -VE ENERGY STATE!

Unconsciously self-talking negatively draining your energy, affecting & depleting your self-love. **-ve**

No self-appreciation & self-love increases the chances of dis-ease stresses, exhaustion & illnesses. **-ve**

Constant giving to others & people pleasing, expecting in return can only bring disappointment. **-ve**

Holding on to beliefs that limit you or serve others bringing you further away from your truth. **-ve**

Living the story others have created of you, consuming you, your mind & your 'One' life. **-ve**

What decisions have you made that caused your life to change?

My most significant decision happened when I realised that the person my two boys had chosen as a female role model, was me. I was a representative of their future female partner, companion and team member.

This knowledge stopped me in my tracks. I was a too-sensitive, indecisive, overwhelmed woman who struggled with the simplest of tasks. This way of living wouldn't serve anyone and would create an unhealthy existence, leading to more problems. It was vital, for the sake of my boys and myself, to choose differently.

That day created changes in every aspect of my life, from where I was living, to who I was surrounding myself with, to my daily habits. And most powerfully, it changed what I was saying and thinking about myself. This didn't happen overnight. It took time and small, incremental steps in a new and different direction, away from the pain and dis-ease of my mind and body, so I could get closer to my truth.

Of course, my transformation shifted all of our lives, but I realised the benefits of this decision would be beneficial and empowering in the long term and also gave me permission to take more extraordinary actions. It was a powerful lesson to my boys that each one of us is worthy of creating our own life.

What are you passionate about?

Living with guts, intensity and deliberateness.

I really am passionate about living with purpose, in the present, moment by moment.

I adore the idea of love and express this in the way I think, what I do, how I feel and the way I speak. I've finally come to a place in my existence where I feel comfortable with who I am, a unique being with unique wants and desires.

I remember sitting on a plane about four years ago, heading to Melbourne for work. As I'd done pretty much every day of my life, my mind started spinning. What if I get things wrong? What if I make mistakes? What will people think?

As you can tell, I lived in constant doubt about who I was. Then, as I was flipping through the *Qantas* magazine, I came across an interview with Dawn French. It was a short spread, with maybe ten questions about her life and what inspired her. To be honest, all I really remember was how personal all of the questions were and how each word seemed to resonate with self-awareness. Every sentence had a feeling and energy behind it. Even if it reflected vulnerability, it still had an essence of knowing.

This made me stop and think. If someone had asked these questions of me, I would've had no idea how to answer, because I had no knowledge of who I was, which was really how I felt most of my life; somewhat overlooked with no real point.

This was indeed the moment I realised the importance of asking myself the right questions to find out who I actually was. So over the next few years, I did extensive research to get a real understanding of my true self.

With time, effort and action, I came to this place of immense appreciation of who I am and where I've come from. This journey has gotten me to a place of embracing all of the crazy different parts of me, and I've chosen to stand up for who I am, no matter what.

From accepting and embedding these new insights about my importance in this world, and that there's a reason for my existence, came the truth that everyone has this same right. I began to feel my purpose, which is sharing that I have a special place on this earth and a journey to embrace.

Listen to yourself. Hear and understand what you're saying, feeling and doing, so you can know who you are, and more importantly be the person you want to be! As a coach, I recommend this to my clients, as well as friends and family. The most profound and essential job you have is getting to know yourself wholeheartedly and loving the true you.

What an exciting concept!

What do you think are the biggest problems people face in life?

Through my experiences, especially around my self-exploration, I believe that one of the most significant problem people face in life, and I'm speaking from experience, is how we treat ourselves.

On a daily basis, people are unconsciously putting a lot of effort into making sure others are happy, hoping they will do the same. This, unfortunately, takes our time and effort away from what matters, which is taking note of how we like and treat ourselves.

Expectations can consume us and cause us to forget to look after ourselves first, even before our children. A powerful question to ask ourselves is, *Why do I put others first?*

These efforts we put into human kindness and compassion need to start with ourselves. I'm not referring to being selfish but living in a considerate way. It's only when we think about who we are, what we want, what makes us happy, what drives us and what serves us, that we can be anything of value to anyone else.

If we consistently live for others, hoping they also live for us, we'll become exhausted, wasting our precious energy on what we can't control. This also gives us the belief that others are responsible for our happiness or needs.

Learning about our desires, and embracing that they're valid, is essential. More importantly, once we apply effort into being an authentic version of ourselves and stop putting our expectations on others, we might find that they'd been feeling pressured in this role we'd given them without their consent.

This needing to be liked by all, and giving so much to make others happy, creates overwhelming feelings that we're somehow owed something for our efforts.

Please understand that when we expect others to make us feel good or require them to change so we can feel better, it places us in a state of constant disappointment, which again depletes our energy.

How we respond is our responsibility. Expecting others to fix and change us is not a healthy place to be. Instead, we need to start putting our wants and needs in our own hands, which is where our power sits.

We need to take a look at

- what we're doing to fill our needs.
- how we expect people to fulfill our needs and keep getting disappointed.
- how much energy we're wasting seeking love and approval from others.
- where and how we're blaming others through our words and/or actions.
- how we expect others to make us happy.
- our need to be liked.

This is a chance to reflect and be aware of how much we expect others to make us happy and how we keep getting disappointed when they don't live up to our expectations.

Taking the time to look at our truths, and being honest with ourselves, is way up on the self-empowering list. It's vital for surviving in life with strength and endurance. When we hold our truths and take responsibility for our way of thinking, speaking and being, we sit in a harmonious, aligned place.

The minute we consider ourselves first, our energy, the way we speak and what we do, will come from a loving, respecting place, rather than a drained, disappointed one.

What's the best way to help them with this problem?

This is a big concept for many, because throughout life, we're taught to look out for and think of others, and definitely not to spend time sitting in our own bubble. When we begin to realise the power of caring for ourselves and building our inner strength, is when we can give more from an honest place. We'll no longer put our expectations on others, because we're fulfilling our own needs and coming from a place of giving.

So the first thing we need to do is write, speak and believe a new story around ourselves and the importance of who we are. This shift may take some time if you've never seized the opportunity to discover your unique story, which only happens when you use the words and actions that resonate with you and represent how you want to live.

This means the key to learning about who we are, is doing so with compassion and self-kindness!

We need to tap into what we truly want and slowly do more of what serves us. Once we do, the rest becomes more manageable. There are many ways to start, but the most valuable is to take time for ourselves. This includes nurturing ourselves on as many levels as possible.

When I realised that I needed to think about me, my health and my understanding of myself, I took the time to choose a new environment and points of view that made more sense. I joined workshops and courses, and I searched for guidance through mentors and coaches who resonated with me. It allowed me to feel safe sharing, knowing I would be free from judgment.

After a while, I also began to value the concept of getting quiet with myself. I took the time to learn to meditate and slowly train myself to imagine who I wanted to be and what I wanted to stand for. I embedded gratitude for my life and my self-power, and began to embrace and feel pride around the changes I decided to make.

Every little step got me closer to a place where I felt good about who I actually was, what I stood for and my right to be me. By shifting the energy around myself, and feeling more centred every day, I began the journey of growing my self-worth.

I hope you're beginning to see the power of your choices. Check in with yourself and ask the following questions:

- What am I saying to myself?
- What identity am I portraying?
- What are the beliefs I'm holding onto that others may have created?
- Is what I'm saying about myself serving me?

Pay attention to your thoughts and beliefs. If they are serving you, make them stronger and louder in every way. If not, do what you can to correct them, and start with a new self-conversation. Be kinder and gentler with yourself.

Live with meaning! Get honest. Make improving your beliefs about yourself, and what's holding you back, a priority.

The good news is that this effort gets easier and more beneficial the more you decide you're worth it.

What is the best advice you could give these people?

Every morning, wake up and take a deep, conscious breath, knowing this new day is your chance to live the unlimited story of your one and only life.

Your life is in your power. You get to live in a way that suits you, which may not necessarily be how others choose to live theirs. Look within yourself, and see who you're waking up as and who you're being. This will be evident when you become aware of your thoughts and the words you're repeating, all of which create how you feel.

What story are you holding around yourself? Are you expressing how disorganised you are? Or how late you always are? Or the amount of pain you suffer with? Maybe you continuously complain about how you have trouble sleeping? Do you describe yourself as not confident or that you have a difficult time meeting people? Do you always list your regrets or all you resent? Do you repeat all of the things you don't like about yourself?

All of this, and much more, tends to be what most people concentrate on, so they wind up sending out negative vibes. Become more aware of what you spend your time saying to yourself and others. What's being repeated unconsciously in your mind? Take note. Write it all down, so you can see it.

Every word, every phrase, every repetitive statement you think and share, has an energetic hold on you. How different would you feel and be if you embedded a diversity of positive images that represented you?

If you embrace that you're in control and have permission to rewrite the chapters of your own life, you will begin to feel better about yourself.

Regardless of what you've unconsciously thought or have been told by others regarding who you are, begin to actively change those words and thoughts, and create a new identity.

Imagine feeling, thinking, living and being a different story, existing in a diverse tapestry of positive images, instead of the character traits you've attached to yourself. For example:

- I am decisive.
- I am organised.
- I have a healthy, strong body.
- I sleep peacefully every night.
- I make decisions easily.
- I like who I am becoming.
- I am proud of my choices.
- I am important.

Holding these phrases with desire and intent will incredibly affect your energy, body and mind. This awareness will allow you to consciously be in control of the story you're living. I'm living proof that rewriting, repeating and embedding this energetically with intense, loving and grateful feelings, can only make your existence better.

Over time, you've listened to the negative words you've said about yourself and have been placed on you by others, until you begin thinking and believing they're a hundred percent true.

But let's be honest. They're just habits and concepts you've gotten yourself trapped into, so you have every right to change them. And when you do, your energy and feelings change.

Become more A.W.A.R.E. of the story you're holding onto so tightly:

- **A**cknowledge that you have a right to love and live for you.
- **W**ake-up knowing every brand-new day is yours to live your way.
- **A**ppreciate the choices you're making and how they're changing you.
- **R**epeat the right words and stories consciously, until a better belief has occurred.
- **E**mbrace and engage in your own vision of your life that aligns with who you want to be.

> "Take the time to SHIFT from the old you that believed the negative words, and LIFT into a new you that chooses to SHINE brightly."

What does love mean to you?

The very essence of love is significant within my heart, but just as importantly, in my mind.

Since I built value around myself, I now make sure I feel, think and speak about love as often as possible. I'm deliberate in holding this energy space of love.

> "With love, anything is possible."

I will clarify that I'm talking about love as an energy. I feel power through the words, thoughts, actions and beliefs I share. There's a sense of humility and a gentleness around sitting in compassion and care in all I do. Whether it's walking on the beach or talking with a good friend, I'm embracing the ambience with love and appreciation.

Whenever I speak to myself and others, I make sure I do it from a space of love. And if I choose to spend my precious time either doing activities I enjoy or finishing up my to-do list, I deliberately complete my tasks with a feeling of love and appreciation.

I find ways to look at circumstances differently, so my love energy rises. When I think about and surround myself with an awareness of love, life seems to offer better opportunities and different circumstances. And when life provides growth situations that seem overwhelming and difficult, I make time to treat myself kindly and to look, feel and speak out of love. It helps me get through these times in a smoother way, with less intense emotions.

We all know heavy emotional turmoils can take over and make us feel worse. But if we're able to pause and reflect, it helps us find our inner power and learn from these situations. It allows us to see a gracious, loving side to all we experience. It removes blame, defuses disrespect and lessens judgement for ourselves and others.

> "The force behind uplifting, embracing and accepting love energy is so vast, it would take a lifetime to express."

We see it with animals and how they appreciate and love unconditionally, no matter their circumstances. Or with plants when they flourish, because they're nurtured and cared for. Experiments with water have been done by Masaru Emoto. If words of love are expressed to the water and then frozen, the water droplets crystallise into stunning symmetrical shapes representing peace, rather than distorted, misaligned shapes that represent chaos.

Dr Leonard Horowitz discovered that the wavelength of love is 528Hz, which has been used to heal and change cell structures, DNA and even physical aspects of the world. In 2010, a study in Vancouver stated that 528Hz was used to purify water from the Gulf of Mexico after the massive oil leak.

Most importantly, it helps with children's inner contentment, which thrives when they're raised in a loving environment. It changes their energy, state of being and health. And then when they reach adulthood, they have a balanced sense of themselves.

Therefore, I firmly believe that love in all forms, and in all areas of life, is worth holding onto and feeling as often as possible. Maintaining a loving space, where we forgive and are gentle with ourselves, while sharing love abundantly as much as possible, has such an impacting effect on every aspect of our lives, that it ripples out to all areas.

"The power of love energy is limitless."

This is why it's vital to decide you're worth loving. You need to get to a comfortable place where you're gaining love from yourself.

How can people become their own success story?

I've learned that we can either let life run us, or we can choose to run our own lives.

In creating your life story, remember the five C's.

1. **C**ontain your power
    Monitor where you use your power, from the words you use, to the feelings that come up and the beliefs you're holding onto.

2. **C**onsider the meaning
    Check in with the real you, not the identity you thought was you or made up for you. Make sure your words, feelings and beliefs are valid and benefit YOU!

3. **C**heck what you're holding onto
    Are your beliefs one-hundred-percent true, or is it possible they're just made up? Do these ideas align with who you want to be, or are you letting others decide for you?

4. **C**onsent is key
    Give yourself permission to reflect on these thoughts and beliefs. Choose what to keep, what to let go of and what to rewrite.

5. **C**hoose who you want to change into
    Come up with your new story. Then embrace it, love it and commit to it.

Creating your new self-success story is your right. You're worth the journey of this discovery and to live authentically as you, not as someone others think you are.

"When you grasp the concept of living authentically, you will realise you have your life, love and being in your own hands."

It's all so exciting and energising!

Every time you place your valuable energy into feelings and thoughts that don't work for you, including negative self-talk, harsh conversations and draining beliefs, you deplete your energy. These stories do not serve you and rob your power of living your best life. They take away your strength and affect your health, relationships and successes.

> "Measure how important your life is, and make the necessary changes that will save your inner energy."

How can people change their story?

This is where your journey to finding out about yourself and changing your story begins.

With your self-talk altered to a more powerful, beneficial state, you will view yourself in abundance. Enjoy getting to know yourself and loving and cherishing yourself as your own best friend.

You can get started by answering these questions:

1. What is your favourite colour? How does it make you feel, and why is it important to feel that way?

2. What pastime captures your total attention, where time just disappears?

3. If you could spend today doing what you desire, what would it be? Why?

4. What do you talk about doing the most, but haven't done yet?

5. Which people in your life inspire you, and why?

6. How do you believe people see you? What story are you attached to because of others?

7. How do you feel when you accomplish one of your goals?

8. In what areas of your life do you feel you have your own back?

9. Recall one fantastic day in your life. How were you feeling? Why was it important?

10. When have you felt most empowered, and why?

How does someone keep inspired on a daily basis?

I understand that all of these ideas may make you feel uncomfortable, because they're outside of your usual way of living. However, if you're experiencing small glimpses or full-on movie reels of overwhelm, lack of assuredness and ill health, these are all indicators that you're not living in sync with your true self and are most likely trying to live for others. These feelings, or body concerns, are extreme signs that it's time to make some major changes.

If I hadn't stopped to pay attention to my years of constant aches, stresses, sadness and struggles, I could only imagine where I would be right now. I might not have been able to raise my boys. I came to a massive truth that I had to do something for me. Yes, it took effort, but these actions were necessary for my survival.

With time, I grew to understand and embrace that I was worth the effort of working on myself and that it had to include a whole lot of loving self-nurturing throughout the different processes.

"Loving yourself means loving all of you; being the best you means considering all of your needs."

These are some important questions to ask yourself:

- Do I need to slow down and quiet my mind through meditation?
- Do I need to change my story and envision different possibilities?
- Can I look at myself with acknowledgement and gratitude, so I can shift the words and messages I tell myself?
- Can I absorb nature and all it offers, so I'm able to ground and centre myself more often, and more easily cope with a difficult situation when the need arises?

Why not embrace the idea of feeling like you're on top of things, and nurture yourself through energy-saving habits?

For my own peace of mind, I need to control the stories that can easily spin around me. By following the five C's, I feel empowered and able to embrace my life.

I refer to them often to make sure I come back to me. I control my energy through the words I use to encourage myself to keep going, the feelings I choose to spend time in and the way I live my life.

I sit in peace when I stop and bring all of my energy inwards. I come back to my breath and make time to centre myself.

The most important time to consciously pause and take time for you is when you're feeling out of tune, and your reactions and self-talk are off-track.

> "Go to a place where you feel peaceful. List all of the changes you've embraced that are fulfilling you. Then let your mind wander off to happy moments with friends and family, embracing good times with laughter and love, and appreciating your wondrous, healthy life."

These incredible habits, singularly or combined, will shape how you picture yourself. Making them a part of your new lifestyle alters what you talk about and how you describe your life, and eventually centres your energy on what counts. Hint: it's *you*.

Life is not about the lists, or the traffic, or the demands from others, but what matters to you.

The more you embrace these new visions of your life, and the phrases that play in your mind and heart, the easier your inner world aligns.

You'll be free from the stories that restrict you.

You have the power.

Imagine living in a place where all of your conversations, messages and choices are yours, and you're actually creating more great states of energy, all aligned with your true be-ing.

Embrace your one life. Make it count, because you matter.

Congratulations on getting to know yourself. It's worth the journey!

Begin here with practicing self-kindness and self-love. Free yourself from self-judgement, shame and criticism. Gently create and rewrite the words you share, the messages you send and the feelings you focus on. This journey of altering your beliefs around yourself gets you closer and stronger, to a place where you can consider building healthier boundaries and knowing your soul rights. It puts you in a place where you value your own time and energy.

What are you waiting for?

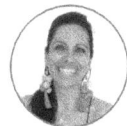

To discover more about how Veronica can help you *Elevate Your Energy*, simply visit www.elevatebooks.com/energy

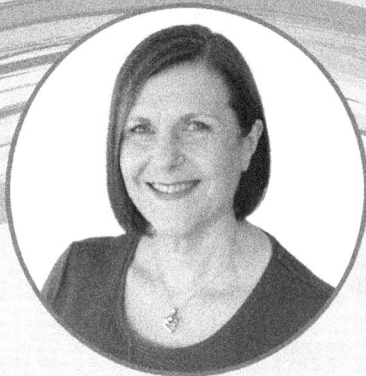

Karen Morley

A Pregnant Pause

Karen Morley is a best-selling author, life coach, Calmbirth® prenatal educator and practitioner in both Resource Therapy (RT) and The Richards Trauma Process (TRTP).

Karen began her professional life as a registered nurse and midwife, before turning her passion to health education and inspiring wellbeing through the mind-body connection.

Her expertise in pre-conception care helps Karen facilitate parents-to-be in preparing for all stages of pregnancy, which includes reducing their fears about conception and childbirth, so they can create a welcoming and nurturing space for their new life in a less-stressful atmosphere.

Karen's capacity for compassion and empathy makes her the ideal practitioner to assist people during their journey from IVF, to pregnancy, birth and beyond.

Karen Morley

A Pregnant Pause

> A pregnant pause is defined as "a silence full of potential
> in the way a pregnant body is full of a new human being.
> A pregnant pause leaves the listener full of anticipation, just like
> a pregnancy is full of excitement about the forthcoming baby."

What are you passionate about?

I trained as a nurse and found my passion in midwifery forty years ago. I loved supporting pregnant people throughout their journey into parenthood.

I'm passionate about assisting others to understand they're enough, and that they're able to shine in the world, while having the satisfaction of knowing they've made a difference.

During my pursuit of nurturing human growth, I found that some of those who attempted conception and IVF, soon discovered it wasn't so easy to conceive.

There was heartache and incessant mind chatter about being prepared or good enough. They would constantly think, *What's wrong with me?* They were made to feel 'less than' for not being able to conceive or were stuck in a cycle of infertility and not knowing how to move out of it. This situation motivated me to provide opportunities for healing and mind-body preparation for conception, pregnancy and beyond. I wanted them to know they were in the best space for handling whatever outcome arose.

Elevate Your Energy

I believe in the right of every person to have the opportunity to grow, nurture and nourish new life, unencumbered by the past and the deep subconscious beliefs that aren't serving them.

I'm passionate about pregnancy, childbirth and making a difference. My goal is to assist those who are struggling to conceive and on their IVF path, to be in a space of peace and calm, rather than fear and anxiety.

What is the best thing that has ever happened to you, and why?

The learning and joy my family awakened in me as they entered my world, inspired me to appreciate the little things and the wonder of nature.

After birthing and nurturing my three beautiful girls, I loved seeing them grow into magnificent women, who themselves became mothers of wonderful children. I was present at their births and am now blessed with nine grandchildren and one on the way.

What is your big WHY?

My children and grandchildren are my biggest Why. I want to be an example and shine brilliantly by being who I was created to be, and doing so without fear or trepidation.

I want to make a difference in the lives of people I encounter each and every day, so they feel secure in their authenticity and are unencumbered by past hurts and distress.

What is the worst thing that has ever happened to you, and how did you overcome it?

When I married my second husband, my dear friend from school, it was a dream come true. My eldest daughter was twelve, and the youngest was seven. We were so excited about embarking on this journey together.

I was passionate about extending our family to encompass the children we'd conceive together, so my happiness increased when I discovered I was pregnant. But my excitement was soon dashed after experiencing miscarriage after miscarriage.

The fifth time, I was monitored closely by the specialist obstetrician. Everything was on track, so we embarked on a short holiday together with the girls.

On our way home, I went to the obstetrician for an ultrasound. Following this visit, my husband and I were going to tell the girls we were expecting. I was watching the screen, so excited that at last, this baby would join us.

Then the obstetrician paused as he gently indicated where the heart was. I didn't comprehend at first. And then it hit me. The little heart wasn't beating as it should. I was admitted to hospital to have a curette.

Instead of a happy conversation, there was a sad one in its place.

I look back now and realise that I was headed into a depression that was insidious and would affect my life and my being.

I did not make good choices.

I contemplated IVF but felt defeated and decided to stop before embarking on the process, accepting for the moment that I wasn't going to continue along this path. I wanted to know more and to understand how I could have helped prepare my body in the most optimal way to nurture a growing baby. I was moving through a greater depth of understanding the process of birth and the evolution of a family.

This led me to studying and learning about the body and the cycles a woman experiences. It's so powerful and wonderful how our body provides signals throughout our cycles that enable us to heal and nurture ourselves appropriately. I studied natural fertility management and preparation for conception, and also became an aromatherapist, all to support the process for other women.

I noticed that the education and information that's provided in hospitals regarding pregnancy, was more about pain relief and the physical process of labour. I was looking for a solution that wasn't clinical. I sensed there was a spark inherent in everyone, something untapped, that could be ignited. I felt that each person already possessed a toolkit of skills and just needed guidance to access it. This knowing led me to Calmbirth.

I then furthered my education in the healing of the subconscious mind to support women and their families. It was amazing learning about how the brain is 'plastic', and the changes that can be made for the better.

What do you think people's biggest problems in life are?

Not acknowledging how they're an amazing human, with gifts and talents others can appreciate and also grow from.

They allow other people's opinions, actions and thoughts to take precedence in determining their own value and worth in the world, and don't understand the impact that holding past distress and trauma can have physically on the body.

What's the best way to help them with this problem?

Someone experiencing these thoughts and feelings might ask what else can be done that they haven't already tried. They may not understand why this is happening or fear there's something wrong with them. They're desperate to become a parent and believe their time is running out. These thoughts constantly invade their mind space, making it difficult for them to think of anything else.

I help people work through their grief and loss, heal past distress and create a mind-body connection that supports optimal health and functioning. A personalised treatment plan is created for learning neurological balancing and skills, so they're supported as they prepare for conception and the IVF process.

Holding their space with care and respect, while being fully present, are vital steps to nurturing people in sessions, either in person or via Zoom, where their emotional pain can be safely explored and integrated.

They need to know that they're enough and have all they need to live their life with meaning, passion, love and joy.

It's important for them to shift their unconscious core beliefs (UCBs) that are driving their current actions and have an impact on their physical and mental wellbeing.

Having consistent, supportive mechanisms that work for them is essential for nurturing and nourishing themselves to be the best person they're designed to be.

Routines and creative endeavours can exponentially expand their current way of being.

What is your biggest life lesson?

To be true to myself and not become what I think others are expecting me to be. This includes accepting what's happened in the past and not allowing it to define me.

I came to understand where I was stuck, what blocks were holding me back and how to heal these areas.

I figured out how my body responds to all of these negative experiences and thoughts, whether consciously or subconsciously, and how they influence my outcomes in ways that don't always support me.

I've learned over time that I was like a willow that would bend and move according to the needs of others, and in doing so, I also missed the opportunity to learn more about who I was uniquely becoming and evolving into.

If you were speaking to your younger self, what advice would you give?

Stop and be silent. Breathe and listen to that still, small voice that has the ultimate wisdom and guidance.

Befriend that voice, and come to know that it's wise. Just let it speak to you, and follow the advice given.

The noise of others giving their advice, and the sound of your own worry telling you what you "should" do, are often loud. Acknowledge them and then put them aside. Ask your inner wisdom for clear guidance and direction.

Be gentle with yourself, and know that everything that happens to you isn't always because of you, so reach out when you're in need of help.

Trust your instinct to choose those who will assist you in the best possible way for what you need at that time. You can overcome the distress and trauma of past experiences that are impacting on your present. It can be released, so you can move on and open your body to its amazing ability to support you.

How would you like to be remembered?

For being a kind, caring, supportive and loving person who only saw the best in others.

I want to be remembered for working with women and couples on their journey to building a family and know I made a difference in their lives. I would like a smile and a peacefulness to enter the spirit of the person remembering who I was, and to have joy expand their heart.

What would you like your legacy to be?

My children, grandchildren, and all who follow, having tremendous love for themselves and others, with a complete knowing of the path they're taking and a willingness to listen and be truly present with others.

I hope I've taught them to know when they can reach out and offer a hand, and also when to step away or just be still.

My legacy is about women throughout the world understanding that they have so much to offer and are role models for their children, with their wisdom and skills. I want to pass down the knowledge that once they've healed their past trauma, they can be free to grow and nurture children, and influence generations to come.

What is the one message you wish to share with the world?

Believe that you have a gift in yourself to share. No matter what's happened in your past, you can begin anew. You are a diamond. Allow yourself to shine and influence others. Let your mind and body come back into balance, so you can heal, and all possibilities can be realised.

What do you think is your life purpose?

My purpose is to be open and shine with love, light, peace and joy. It's my mission to let others know the truth of who they are and the difference they make in people's lives for the greatest good.

All I want is to help alleviate the distress and trauma that resides within, so everyone can let go and heal. Also, supporting those who wish to conceive, no matter the method, on their journey.

What do you believe you've been put on the planet to do?

To be kind, caring, supportive and present, while gently allowing people to know what's possible for themselves.

I have an image of myself as a beautiful stone dropped gently into a still pond. The ripples expand out from the point of contact, ever growing and expanding, reaching so many more people than I could ever have known possible.

How are you currently making a difference in people's lives?

When I'm with someone, I'm completely present, holding them gently and with care in a safe space. I inspire those embarking on a journey of change to have trust in themselves that they are enough.

Through Calmbirth prenatal education, Resource Therapy (RT), The Richards Trauma Process (TRTP) and Results/Life Coaching, I'm helping individuals overcome the loops of anxiety, depression, fear and unhelpful patterns, to make different choices with a new mind frame.

I show those who are anxious and stressed how to come back to being calm and present within themselves.

They allow their bodies to heal their subconscious drivers, so they can have peace.

Have you had any aha moments that changed everything for you?

I came to realise that what another person projects onto me, is really about their own hurt and pain.

Calmbirth tapped into the power that was already present in me. It enabled me to show people what they had in a focused way, so they could use it in their life, in pregnancy, during birth and beyond.

Attending and supporting my friends and children's partners at the birth of their babies, provided me with a fuller, richer understanding of the process. It gave me an opportunity to support them, which turned out to not only be foundational in them becoming a family, but further developed and enriched my skills of being a passionate Calmbirth practitioner.

What decisions have made a difference in your life?

I wanted to continue my exploration of midwifery and facilitating prenatal education with couples and single people alike. I enjoyed creating a welcoming and empowering space for those embarking on the birth experience, but I knew there was so much untapped power that could be unleashed.

Witnessing people caught in distress, rumination, habitual thoughts and actions that caused blockages, led me to further training in Resource Therapy and The Richards Trauma Process. They provided more pieces of the puzzle in my understanding of healing past distress and trauma that can disrupt optimal functioning of the body.

How did you become interested in mindset?

I would always bend, shape-shifting into who I thought others wanted me to be, so I could be accepted. Instead of finding myself, I became more and more lost, uncertain and unclear about who I uniquely was. I came to realise that this was unfair to my partners. If I couldn't appreciate or express myself, how could they ever know the real me?

When I began studying mindset, it changed how I viewed the world. I could be open to the differences in others, and also grow to understand more about myself. It was an exciting time of discovery. I stepped into my fear of the unknown and was surprised by the discoveries along the way. I was particularly excited to know that thoughts and your network of neurons could be altered and weren't fixed in stone.

Hope became my beacon, and I was attracted to it like a moth to a flame.

There was one more thing I needed to learn that would weave all of the skills and training together, and provide a holistic outlook. That was life coaching.

It provided me an avenue to explore even more deeply how our brain can change, and the unlimited possibilities of how one person could make a difference.

What's the biggest mistake people make in the area of mindset?

Ignoring the importance of the mind-body connection and the way the body holds onto past distress and trauma, which in turn influences its biochemistry and neurological functioning. The mind has a tremendous impact on the body, and the subconscious drives all functions, so they must be in accord to provide a healthy environment for a baby to be conceived.

They don't realise that it's not only the body that may be causing difficulties in conceiving. It may be the core beliefs being held within the subconscious mind.

Also, being swayed by other people's opinions, actions and thoughts.

Consumed with wanting to please others, they'll join a group that doesn't reflect who they are or their own values. They'll become a chameleon, adapting to be acceptable within this environment, without ever questioning or determining what's important to them.

Do you feel mindset is important?

It's the direction in which we need to head. It's the rudder directing the sailboat of our lives.

Mindset is so very important and an often-overlooked area when it comes to pregnancy or infertility.

The mind is divided into two parts: the conscious, which is what we're aware of, and the subconscious, which is below our conscious thought.

The conscious mind is where willpower, long term memory, and logical and critical thinking come from. It can support us in creating change and making a difference, but it has its limits. Have you ever wondered why possessing all the willpower in the world doesn't help with weight loss, bad habits or addictions, those nagging thoughts, or the symptoms of Post-Traumatic Stress Disorder (PTSD)?

We think our conscious mind is doing everything, but actually, the subconscious is running the show.

The subconscious mind is incredibly faster and far more powerful than the conscious mind. This is why I believe tapping into it and using its amazing capabilities to support us is the key to restoring our wellbeing.

The subconscious is the storehouse of all of our learning, experiences and anything that has ever made an impression on us. It constantly monitors our internal and external world and is where beliefs, habits, values, emotions, protective reactions, long-term memory, imagination and intuition reside. It's what drives all of our electrical impulses and chemical reactions that regulate our bodily functions.

All of this is happening without the help, supervision or engagement of the conscious part of the mind. The beliefs that "I'm not good enough, so I'm not going to be a good parent" or "I'll wait until I'm older to become a parent", whether they're in the conscious or subconscious, can become a block to conceiving.

Beliefs are conclusions that are usually formed at an earlier age and are derived from information and/or experience. They're about how you think and feel, and they, in turn, create your perceptions about life.

Are your current beliefs serving you well?

> "The more we think the same thoughts, which then produce the same chemicals, which cause the body to have the same feelings, the more we physically become modified by our thoughts. In this way, depending on what we are thinking and feeling, we create our state of being."
> ~ Joe Dispenza

What is the stress response?

Beliefs, thoughts and past experiences determine whether we perceive a situation as a threat and thus need to rally the sympathetic nervous system (SNS), responsible for fight/flight/freeze, otherwise known as the stress response.

If we think about it, we're wired to respond to stress and threat, which can be real or imagined. When in this state, the body is not in the best position to nurture a baby within the womb. All of the circulating energy and chemicals are directed to service the parts of the body necessary for protection, rather than providing for a growing baby.

In today's society, thoughts and experiences that are relived, either consciously or subconsciously, keep the body on heightened alert and on standby for action.

Unfortunately, as mentioned above, the stress response can be triggered not only by the environment, but by our thoughts and beliefs. Some of these thoughts may be concerns about

- your pregnancy not happening as quickly or easily as you'd hoped
- finances and not being able to afford the expensive treatments
- your safety
- being 'good enough'
- what might be wrong
- your biological clock
- your digestive system issues
- tension in your relationships
- unresolved distress
- your poor physical health
- your hormonal and reproductive health issues.

All of these thoughts can hinder effective functioning of the body for conceiving, maintaining a healthy pregnancy, having an empowered birth and living as a healthy, happy family unit.

I believe that due to our current lifestyle, there's a huge impact on our health. Our level of stress remains high because of constant, increasing demands regarding caring for others, issues at home, pressures at work and the ongoing interaction with social media.

Some of the physical manifestations of stress in the body can cause

- sleep problems
- depression and/or anxiety
- fatigue/exhaustion
- irritability/mood swings and emotional problems
- sensitivity to light and/or noise
- headaches
- muscle tension or jaw clenching
- shoulder and neck aches, pains and tightness
- racing heart
- high blood pressure
- menstrual irregularities
- thyroid issues
- allergies
- inflammation
- digestive upsets/irritable bowel, bloating, diarrhoea and constipation
- poor immune function
- hormonal imbalances and excessive sweating
- infertility or PCOS, and sometimes uterine fibroids.

Is it any wonder that the reproductive functions are suppressed and/or you develop food intolerances and digestive issues?

There are multiple causes for these symptoms, so it's important to get advice from your healthcare practitioner.

What is the relaxation response?

When we perceive we're in a state of safety, it allows our body to relax, digest, repair and reproduce. This is due to the relaxation response, or the parasympathetic nervous system (PNS), which is responsible for rest and renewal, and the body returning to its natural balance, or homeostasis.

My understanding is that the hormones, or messenger chemicals responsible for the healthy functioning of our reproductive and other systems, primarily belong to the parasympathetic system. They decrease your metabolism, heart rate and breathing, which slows down your brainwaves to enable clearer thinking.

The body needs to have a balance to function optimally. We can retrain our responses and bring forth the relaxation response, a bodily calm that reduces the harmful effects of stress.

What about breathwork?

Breathwork is an invaluable tool that if used with consistency, is a skill that will enhance your overall health and wellbeing, allowing the systems within your body to function well. This can make a critical difference to the success of any other therapy you may undertake.

Connecting the mind and body can be done by slowing the breath and activating the parasympathetic nervous system.

Here are just a few ways you can control your breathing:

- Sit and stand more upright and open with your body.
- Breathe through your nose. Breathing through the mouth stimulates the sympathetic nervous system, preparing you for fight or flight.
- Deepen and slow your breath, and breathe out slightly longer than you breathe in. This can help activate the PNS, because the air inhaled is moistened, filtered and warmed.

Why is it important to develop an awareness of your subconscious state?

Knowing what's surfacing at any given moment gives you the wisdom and power to influence your system in a different way, so you can activate the PNS and bring the body back to a state of balance and harmony.

Stored emotions within the body that aren't consciously remembered, and those that continue to surface and cause havoc, can impact your systems and disturb your equilibrium.

You might say, "I'm meditating and following all of these calming practices. Why am I still not moving forward?"

As I mentioned, the conscious mind isn't aware of what the subconscious mind is doing. We can only gain glimpses through our own reactions, such as having a sense of anxiety or discomfort, repeating habits that aren't serving you, saying things that seem to come out of nowhere and overreacting.

Unwanted feelings can surface, such as

- panic attacks
- fears
- phobias

- anxiety
- a sense of worthlessness or feeling unlovable
- revisiting or having flashbacks of traumatic or disturbing events.

You may experience unwanted behaviours, including

- addictions
- disordered eating
- compulsiveness.

There could also be unwanted thoughts, such as

- ruminating
- feeling depressed or in despair, with no energy to do anything.

All of these are long-buried in the subconscious and should cause concern. They can have an impact on the chemicals and hormones that control your body and hold you in a stress response.

We can't usually control our SNS with our conscious thought, but there are strategies that can calm the mind and bring the system into a more balanced state.

Exercising or taking a short walk when you feel stress coming on, or taking stock of what you've accomplished throughout the day and what you're grateful for, are a couple of strategies that can help.

When you work with me, we follow a dynamic, rich and sequenced process that resolves distressing events and issues, such as anxiety, depression, fears, phobias and extreme trauma, quickly, effectively and safely. I always allow space for your needs to be met, and you will be treated with care and respect.

Also, I would never require detailed remembering or rehashing of past distressing or traumatic events.

How can Resource Therapy help?

Resource Therapy was founded and developed by Dr Gordon Emmerson. It's an empowering therapy based on the understanding that our personality is made up of many parts, called our Resources, that are available to us. They can work for us or be disruptive, causing distress, unwanted behaviours or conflict. These issues can be treated and resolved in a fraction of the time spent using some other therapies that speak only to the conscious and not where the issue originates, in the subconscious, which means there's longer-lasting change.

Resource Therapy brings the part of the personality that needs change into the conscious, so that it can be worked with directly, which frees it to help you resume positive functions.

Therefore, there's likely hidden parts of you that can come to the surface in a healthy way and back you up when needed. Once you identify these resources, they can assist your entire self, where before it might have seemed impossible.

> "We are born with all of the resources we will ever need."
> ~ *Virginia Satir*

Could you explain The Richards Trauma Process (TRTP)?

Judith Richards has an intimate understanding of trauma. It led her to create The Richards Trauma Process (TRTP), which teaches that there is a way to the other side of trauma and its myriad symptoms.

TRTP doesn't merely address the symptoms of distress or trauma, it resolves the issues of extreme trauma and is equally as effective in treating lower levels of anxiety, depression, fears and phobias. Pretty much any issue that's trauma-related.

TRTP deals with the underlying cause of the problem, thus removing the emotional charge from the past and returning you to a state of empowerment and calm. The body knows that the events are over, and it's safe. The underlying, unconscious core beliefs that keep you stuck in patterns of thought, emotion and behaviour, are attended to.

Deep imagination is used in order to deal with distress or trauma where it's stored in your subconscious and body, and speaks directly to them. You move from fight/flight/freeze and feeling that you're not safe, to being in an empowered, self-regulated state, and calm returns on all levels. Symptoms cease, and the memory of the distress or trauma is placed firmly in the past.

What is Calmbirth, and how does it help with the pregnancy process?

Calmbirth is quality childbirth education. It's about improving birth outcomes and changing birth culture in Australia. Support is offered once pregnancy is achieved, and you're nurturing your baby.

Peter Jackson, Calmbirth's founder, explains it this way:
Calmbirth does not advocate for one way to give birth. It's about helping couples create a positive birth experience, no matter how that birth unfolds. The program is designed to teach mothers to use their inner resources to work with birth, and to help them understand the process of birth, so they can help the baby into the world, instead of resisting the labour journey.

It's one of the first childbirth education programs to be evidence-based and is clinically and scientifically proven to

- **reduce** the rates of medical intervention
- **reduce** the use of pain relievers and epidurals during childbirth
- **reduce** the impact of perinatal anxiety and postnatal depression after childbirth

▸ **enrich** a woman's birth experience, so it's positive, irrespective of how they give birth.

The Calmbirth program is founded on research from neuroscience, midwifery, obstetrics and epigenetics, and uses an extensive understanding of the relaxation response and its influence on the birthing process. It has unparalleled success in helping birthing women releasing their fear.

It provides an understanding of the mind-body connection and how a woman's emotional state influences the birth, both mentally and physically. The program continues to be updated in collaboration with experts, including a range of birthing, education, parenting and mind-body specialists.

Jane Svensson, Clinical Midwifery Consultant in Health Education at the Royal Hospital for Women, says:

Calmbirth is a program that explores the mind-body connection. How the hormones of pregnancy, and then labour and birth, interact in a synergy that makes the female body infinitesimally able to nurture new life and give birth to a child at whatever stage that it is. Calmbirth's growth and popularity lies in the fact that today's women and couples want to take control of their body and learn how best they can nurture their unborn child, not only in labour, but also in the prenatal weeks. They don't want to be the passive recipient of their care. They want to be active participants. Calmbirth promotes and fosters this.

The focus of Calmbirth is on educating couples on all areas of birth. It provides practical skills and techniques that can be used during birth, in order to empower them to let go of their fear and anxiety, and allows them to have a positive birth experience.

The course outline includes the following:

1. Understanding how your mental state, thoughts and beliefs, leading up to, and on the day of the birth, not only dictates your experience, but also the way your body works with labour and birth.

2. The physiology of birth...how your body gives birth.

3. Tools, techniques and practical skills to assist you mentally and physically.

4. The role of the partner, who is provided with their own 'toolbox'.

5. Preparation for all birth journeys.

6. Conscious parenting and ensuring you're aware of the role you and your baby play in bringing your baby into the world.

What are your tips for getting through a difficult time in life?

- Be aware.
- Be an observer, like a director watching a movie unfold.
- Treat others the way you want to be treated, with care, love and nurturing.
- Have a support team around you.
- Listen without judgment or giving advice, so people feel comfortable being honest with you.
- Establish good sleep/hygiene practices.
- Limit screen time.
- Take a break from social media.
- Only watch entertainment that uplifts and makes you laugh.
- Walk in nature.
- Give long, lingering hugs.
- Hug a tree.
- Walk barefoot on grass or on the beach.
- Breathe in deeply and slowly through your nose.
- Still the mind often.

- Let go with grace what no longer serves.
- Drift to beautiful memories or scenes.
- Appreciate the little things in your life. Have a gratitude journal, and reflect each night about three things you're grateful for.
- Each morning set the intention of how you want to show up.
- Set an hourly reminder to stop, breathe and be grateful for the support that's always there.

What is your most inspiring client story?

I watched one of my clients have the most amazing shift in mindset. It showed on her body and face as she let go of the old stories from a traumatic birth. She healed from within and appeared transformed before my eyes. She went from fear of being pregnant and giving birth, to being relaxed and present, truly knowing that she could work with her body to birth her baby, however it would unfold.

How do you help people with their healing?

Becoming a family is an amazing opportunity for growth, learning and expanding our knowledge of how we are in the world. As we grow and educate ourselves, we impart this learning to our children and provide a supportive and nurturing environment, so they can flourish and be the best they can be in the world. And when they become parents, they can pass it on. We can impact many generations and make the world a better place.

With care, support and assistance, we're able to recognise how we can change our thoughts, calm our body and be filled with excitement for a new and different way. We'll know that whatever and however everything unfolds, we can feel empowered, with a sense of direction and calm.

These are the ways I can assist you in your healing:

- Understanding your menstrual cycle and what your symptoms indicate.
- Calming the nervous system.
- Getting to know your body and what it's telling you. (Your own healing is there for you.)
- Identifying quality sleep hygiene and the importance of melatonin.
- Reducing blue light and screen time.
- Nourishing the body with wholesome, vibrant and healthy foods.
- Looking after the microbiome of the body and supporting your gut health.
- Moving the body through gentle exercise in nature.
- Being present with yourself and others.
- Nurturing the mind and cultivating habits, thoughts and beliefs that will guide you towards expansion, openness, love and joy.
- Finding time for quiet reflection.
- Hydrating with good quality, healthy water.
- Self-soothing techniques.
- Calming the nervous system for optimal functioning.
- Emotional healing, which allows you to break old patterns that no longer serve you.
- Visualising.

Does visualisation help in life?

I use visualisation often, personally and within my work. It helps those experiencing anxiety to be calm and present, so they're in partnership with their healing.

During my Calmbirth classes, we do a lot of visualising and trusting that we can work with however the process unfolds. I teach how to believe in the power of the body and seeing every part splendidly doing what it's designed to do.

I work with clients to help them see a future as rich as they want it to be.

I also use it to aid my natural healing process and see the outcome I want.

What is your simple formula for health?

- Learn to listen to your body and its signals, and gently provide what it needs to bring it back to optimal health.
- Reach out to others who can help you on your path.
- Be open to learning more about yourself and what nurtures you for your best health outcomes.
- Learn to listen.
- Be open and aware.
- Act with wisdom.
- Seek help when needed.

What are the best ways people can find energy?

- Finish your shower with cold water to activate your immune system.
- Flush your body with filtered, electrolysed, hydrogen-rich water.
- Look after your microbiome and gut health.
- Limit screen time before bed for two hours and when rising in the morning. Let the sun be the first light you see.
- Remain connected through meditation and prayer.
- Have daily interactions with inspiring people.
- Be mindful and present throughout the day.
- Ask for guidance, be still and listen, and then act accordingly.

Use your resources in conjunction with a trusted health care practitioner who can have a positive impact on your outcome.

Take some time to refocus and be present with yourself and the wonder of who you are, so you're refreshed and replenished for whatever lies ahead, however it unfolds. Know that you're enough and in an optimal space to welcome, grow and nurture a baby.

Let's take the first step, and be open to all possibilities.

To discover more about how Karen can help you *Elevate Your Energy*, simply visit www.elevatebooks.com/energy

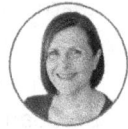

Afterword

While you were reading these people's inspiring stories, did you notice something? All of their life experiences were for a purpose, bringing them closer to their goals, relationships and especially the message they were meant to share with the world.

The last page is a blank canvas for you to write the next chapter of your own story about elevating your energy and inspiring others. Every day is a brand-new opportunity to be the author of your destiny.

Next Steps

To support you on your journey to *Elevate Your Energy,* we recommend you take advantage of these resources:

🖥 7 Day Transformation Program

Learn ONE powerful 'Elevate Process' you can use immediately to improve Your Relationships, Health, Finances, Mindset and any other area of your life.

To join this 7-day transformation online program, simply go to: www.elevatebooks.com/you

👥 Connect with the Authors

To discover more about the authors and what they have to teach you, and bonus gifts they are offering visit:
www.elevatebooks.com/energy

🎙 Subscribe to our Podcast

If you'd like to hear the go-to interviews from the authors and be re-inspired, check out: www.elevatebooks.com/podcast

🌐 Visit the Website

To find out more about the Elevate book series, visit: www.elevatebooks.com